# THE SIRTFOOD DIET

### The Ultimate Guide for a Healthy Weight Loss. Learn How to Boost Your Metabolism, Burn Fat and Lose Weight Easily

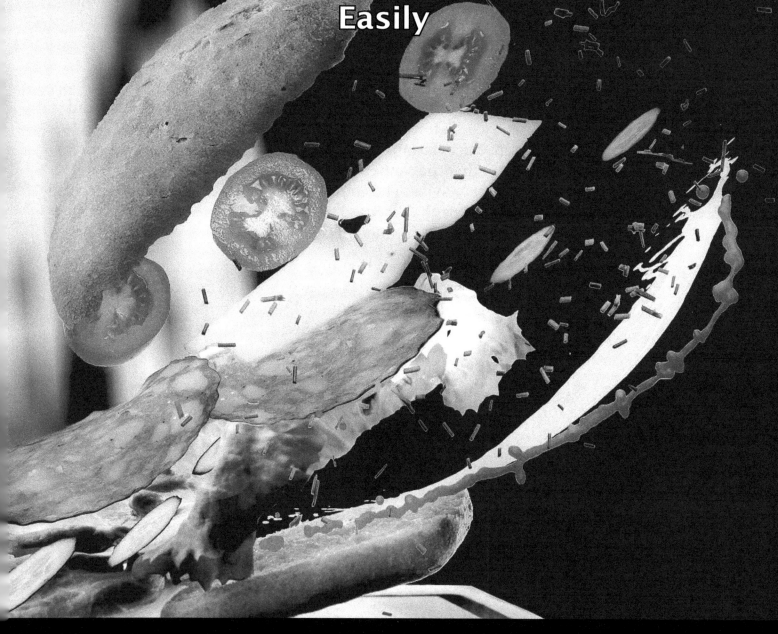

*Copyright - 2020 -*

*All rights reserved.*

The content contained within this book may not be reproduced, duplicated or transmitted without direct written permission from the author or the publisher.

Under no circumstances will any blame or legal responsibility be held against the publisher, or author, for any damages, reparation, or monetary loss due to the information contained within this book. Either directly or indirectly.

*Legal Notice:*

This book is copyright protected. This book is only for personal use. You cannot amend, distribute, sell, use, quote or paraphrase any part, or the content within this book, without the consent of the author or publisher.

*Disclaimer Notice:*

Please note the information contained within this document is for educational and entertainment purposes only. All effort has been executed to present accurate, up to date, and reliable, complete information. No warranties of any kind are declared or implied. Readers acknowledge that the author is not engaging in the rendering of legal, financial, medical or professional advice. The content within this book has been derived from various sources. Please consult a licensed professional before attempting any techniques outlined in this book.

By reading this document, the reader agrees that under no circumstances is the author responsible for any losses, direct or indirect, which are incurred as a result of the use of information contained within this document, including, but not limited to, - errors, omissions, or inaccuracies.

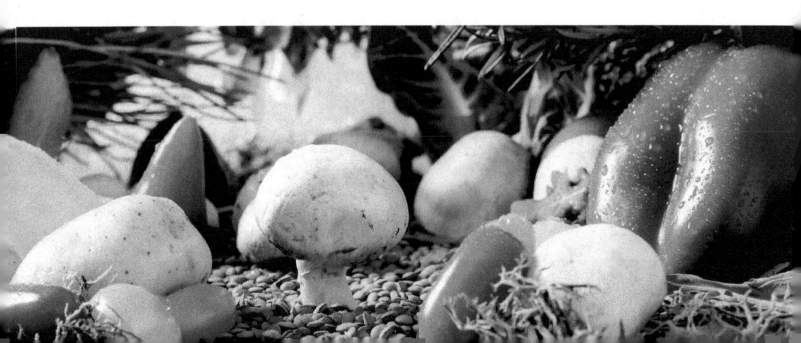

# Table of Contents

| | |
|---|---|
| **INTRODUCTION** | 4 |
| **CHAPTER 01** | |
| Sirt Food Diet Theory | 8 |
| **CHAPTER 02** | |
| How to Activate Your Skinny Gene without Fasting | 14 |
| **CHAPTER 03** | |
| The Scientific Basis of Sirt Diet | 18 |
| **CHAPTER 04** | |
| The Top 20 Sirt Food and Other Ingredient for a Sirt-Full Diet | 22 |
| **CHAPTER 05** | |
| Diet Sirt and Physical Exercise | 26 |
| **CHAPTER 06** | |
| Sirtfoods in Detail | 30 |
| **CHAPTER 07** | |
| Maintaining | 34 |
| **CHAPTER 08** | |
| Shopping List | 40 |
| **CHAPTER 09** | |
| The Sirtfood Green Juices and Smoothies | 46 |
| **CHAPTER 10** | |
| Recipes: | 50 |
| Breakfast | 50 |
| 01 Sirtfood Green Onion and Mushroom Omelet | 51 |
| 02 Sirtfood Nutmeg-coated Creamy French Toast | 52 |
| 03 Dried Cherry and Golden Raisin Turnovers | 53 |
| 04 Sirtfood Muffins | 54 |
| 05 Baked Eggs With Cantal Cheese | 55 |
| **CHAPTER 11** | |
| Recipes: | 56 |
| Salads | 56 |
| 06 Sirtfood Green Salad | 57 |
| 07 Sirtfood Layered Taco Salad | 58 |
| 08 Cucumber Fennel Salad | 60 |
| 09 Sirtfood Apple Coleslaw | 61 |
| 10 Carrot Bean Salad | 62 |
| **CHAPTER 12** | |
| Recipes: | |
| Meat | 64 |
| 11 Sirtfood Pork Roast | 65 |

| | |
|---|---|
| 12 SIRTFOOD FRIED CHICKEN | 66 |
| 13 SIRTFOOD STEAK DIANE | 67 |
| 14 TURKEY SANDWICH | 68 |
| 15 TACO BELL SPICY TOSTADA | 69 |

## CHAPTER 13

RECIPES:

| | |
|---|---|
| FISH | 70 |
| 16 SIRTFOOD CRUSTY FISH FILLETS | 71 |
| 17 GARLIC ANCHOVY LINGUINE | 72 |
| 18 TUNA & BOK CHOY PACKETS | 73 |
| 19 SIRTFOOD CARAMEL COATED CATFISH | 74 |
| 20 NEW ORLEANS STUFFED ARTICHOKES | 75 |

## CHAPTER 14

RECIPES:

| | |
|---|---|
| SOUPS | 76 |
| 21 SIRTFOOD BEEF TORTELLINI SOUP | 77 |
| 22 SIRTFOOD MEAT AND POTATO SOUP | 78 |
| 23 LEEK SOUP | 79 |
| 24 CHICKEN 'N' DUMPLING SOUP | 80 |
| 25 SIRTFOOD SAUSAGE CABBAGE SOUP | 81 |

## CHAPTER 15

RECIPES:

| | |
|---|---|
| SACKS | 82 |
| 26 SIRTFOOD CHEDDAR CRACKERS | 83 |
| 27 HONEY-PEANUT POPCORN | 84 |
| 28 LOVAGE PESTO | 85 |
| 29 SIRTFOOD MAC 'N CHEESE BITES | 86 |
| 30 NORWEGIAN FLAT BREAD | 87 |

## CHAPTER 16

RECIPES:

| | |
|---|---|
| SPREADS AND DIPS | 88 |
| 31 BROWNIE BATTER BEAN DIP | 89 |
| 32 SIRTFOOD ARTICHOKE AND EGG SPREAD | 90 |
| 33 SPINACH AND ARTICHOKE DIP | 91 |
| 34 PINTO BEAN SPREAD | 92 |
| 35 BROWNIE BATTER DIP | 93 |

## CHAPTER 17

RECIPES:

| | |
|---|---|
| VEGETARIAN RECIPES | 94 |
| 36 SIRTFOOD STEAMED ASPARAGUS | 95 |
| 37 SIRTFOOD VEGETARIAN QUINOA AND CHICKPEA BURGER | 96 |
| 38 VEGETARIAN PAD THAI | 97 |
| 39 FARFALLE WITH CAPERS | 98 |
| 40 GRILLED ASPARAGUS AND MUSHROOMS | 99 |

## CHAPTER 18

RECIPES:

| | |
|---|---|
| VEGAN RECIPES | 100 |
| 41 VEGAN BROCCOLI AND RICE CASSEROLE | 101 |
| 42 FRIED RICE PINEAPPLE | 102 |

    43 Sirtfood Oriental Barbecued Pork     104
    44 Rustic French Chicken     105
    45 Traditional apple Sauce     106

# CHAPTER 19
    Recipes:     108
    Desserts     108
    46 Apricot Delight     109
    47 Spice Bars     110
    48 Sirtfood Pretzel Strawberry Dessert     111
    49 Sirtfood Cherry Cheescake Pie     112
    50 Fluffy Orange Gelatin Pie     113

# CHAPTER 19
    Recipes:
    Green Juice     114
    51 Sirtfood Minty Green Juice     115
    52 Sirtfood Persimmon-Mint Magic     116
    53 Sirtfood Pears N' Spinach     117
    54 Sirtfood Protein Green     118
    55 Sirtfood Sunflower Spinach     119

# CONCLUSION     120

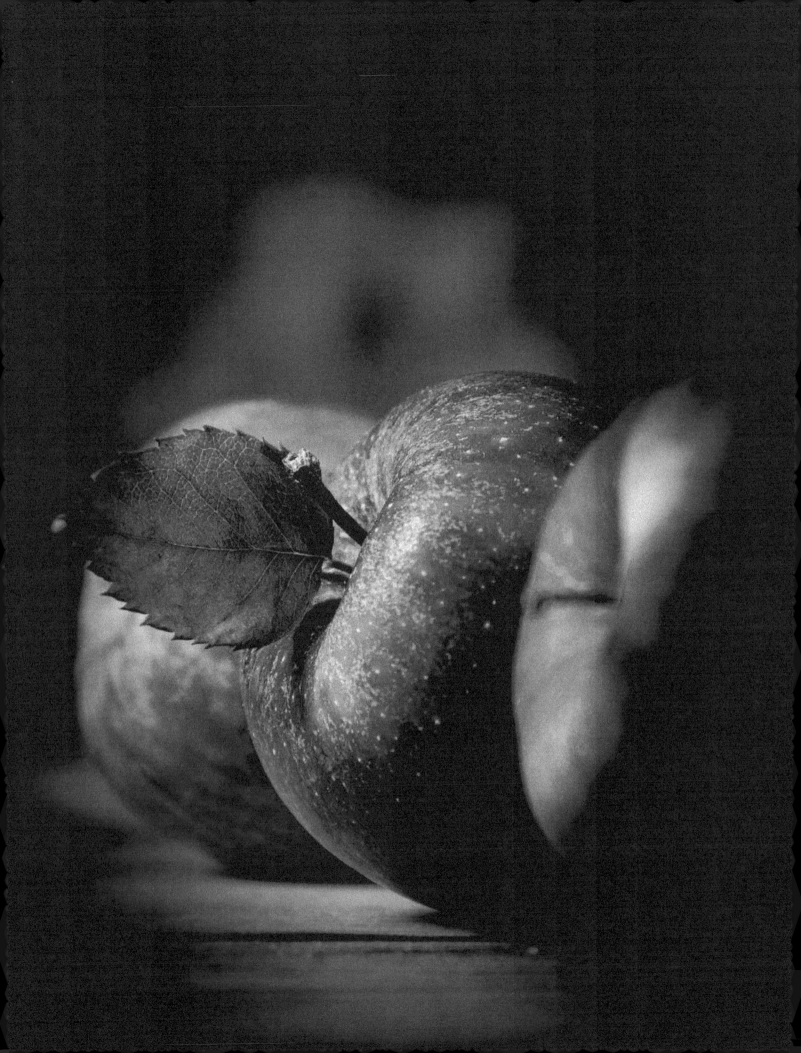

# INTRODUCTION

The Sirt diet takes its name from the fact that it is based on sirtuins, enzymatic proteins that help keep the cells of your body healthy. They allow the regular functioning of our body and protect us from various inflammations.

The originality of the sirt diet leverages the use of foods with particular nutrient molecules, polyphenols, which activate enzymatic proteins, sirtuins. They regulate our metabolism, help us burn fat and obviously make us lose weight.

In reality, the diet has been very well known for some time now, also because several characters from the world of entertainment have decided to try it.

However, it is not only for this reason that it is well known. The obvious weight loss that many people have experienced directly and the fact that it is a diet designed to eat everything, has given even more notoriety. In addition, the diet allows the administration of some of the best foods that nature makes available to us. Dark chocolate 85%, red wine, strawberries and berries make us forget that we are undertaking a diet. In addition to the fact that it is a balanced and healthy diet, you lose weight without losing muscle mass.

The diet was developed by two renowned dietitians in the UK and Ireland, Aidan Goggins and Glen Matten. The two British nutritionists have studied a program according to which a diet based on certain specific foods can promote rapid weight loss and that the lost pounds do not recover. And if you realize you have gained weight, nothing prevents you from starting again. On the other hand, Sirt foods are a guarantee of genuine, fresh and rich in polyphenols, if used in our daily diet.

Losing weight quickly without fatigue is now a reality.

The lean gene diet is an innovative diet. It is based on metabolic regulators, the sirtuins capable of activating a family of genes that exists in each of us. These genes influence our mood, our ability to burn fat and even the mechanisms that regulate our mood and longevity.

The activation of sirtuins, clinically guaranteed by the Sirt diet, produces the same beneficial effects of fasting without the disadvantages. Unlike many other diets, which say what to eliminate, the Diet Sirt says what to add in our nutrition plan during the diet. This is why it is easier to follow than any other diet.

The Sirt diet is a weight loss program that allows you to lose up to 3 kg in a week while staying healthy and fit.

## THE TWO PHASES OF THE DIET

The diet develops in two stages. The initial, more rigid phase lasts one week and involves limiting calories to 1000 kcal for three days. It is allowed to consume a solid meal a day rich in Sirtfood and three green juices.

During phase 1, it is advisable to reduce the caloric intake and to take every day a juice obtained from cabbage, arugula, green apple, parsley, celery stalks and green tea which can be easily made at home with the help of a centrifuge or an extractor. In this first phase it is possible to lose from 3 to 7 kilograms. It is very important to consume around 1000 calories during the first three days.

From the fourth to the seventh day, the heat intake increases to 1500 kcal and includes two green juices and two meals rich in sirtfood per day.

The second phase is known as the "maintenance phase". It lasts 14 days, in which constant weight loss occurs. There are no specific indications regarding the calorie intake, but it is necessary to take a green juice daily and to introduce only Sirt foods in all meals of the day. To maximize results, exercise is also encouraged for about 30 minutes five days a week.

The juices to be made at your choice can include black cabbage, celery, arugula, parsley, green tea and lemon.

Solid meals include turkey, chicken, cabbage curry, prawns, buckwheat noodles and onions. They are all foods that are widely used in the preparation of our daily recipes.

The sirt diet is versatile, open, linked to a natural, healthy and appetizing diet. For vegetarians or vegans there are variants with recipes designed specifically. Sirt juices should be drunk at three different times of the day: on waking up, mid-morning and mid-afternoon. A solid meal is recommended for lunch. Very important is to eat three balanced meals rich in sirtfood per day including a green juice.

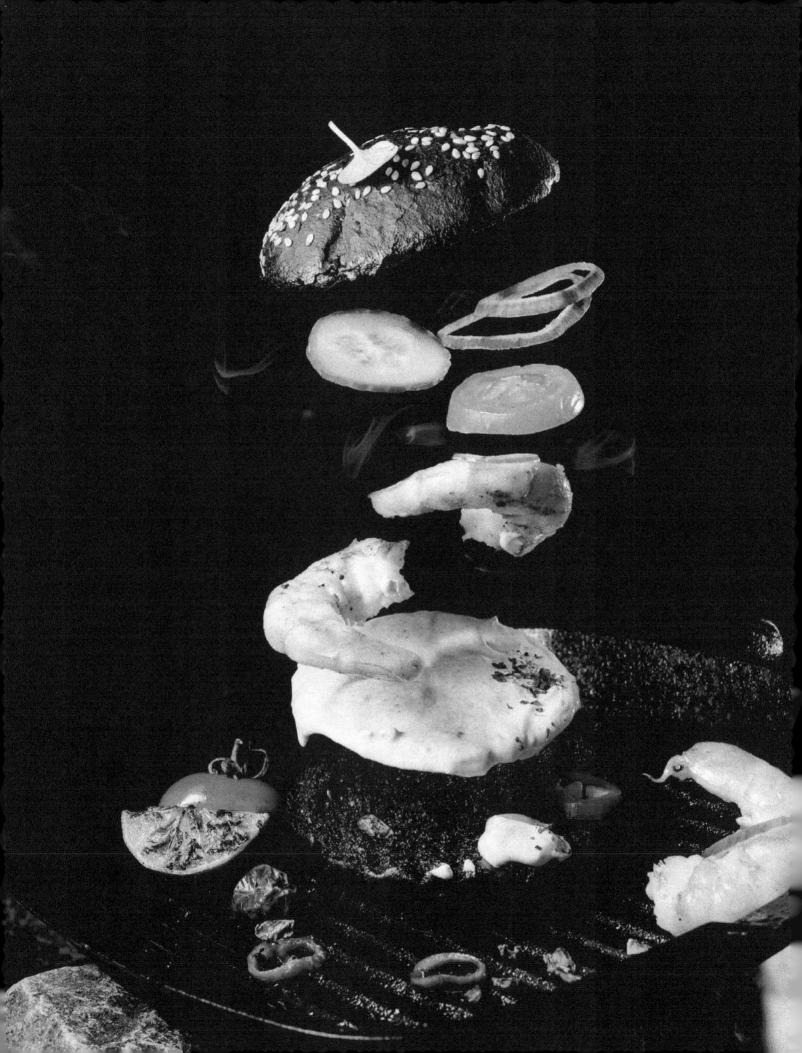

# CHAPTER 01

# Sirt Food Diet Theory

Sirtuins are a class of normally happening proteins in the human body. First found a couple of decades prior, they have energizing capacities, inquire about shows. The explorations were never performed on genuine individuals (selecting rather for test cylinders or lab creatures), however sirtuins have been found to assume a job in clearing free radicals, lessening irritation, managing our inner clock and forestalling maturing. The exploration has persuaded that sirtuins might be utilized to treat or forestall certain infections, like malignant growth and Type 2 diabetes.

It's additionally been discovered that sirtuins might keep fat cells from copying. The proof isn't firm, yet this is the place the "turbo-charge weight loss" guarantee of the Sirtfood Diet originates from.

## THE DIET PLAN

During the initial three days of the diet, you drink two green squeezes and eat only one dinner every day during this time, you are restricted to 1,000 calories for each day. Throughout the following four days, you drink two juices for each day and eat two dinners every day, while constraining yourself to 1,500 calories for each day. After the principal week and for the following 14 days, you expend an abundance of sirtfoods in three dinners and one juice for every day. Following 21 days, the center changes to "Sirtifying" your preferred suppers by embedding or subbing sirtfoods into plans.

Obviously, the advantages of the Sirtfood Diet come rather rapidly. Numerous dieters report significant weight loss and expanded vitality in simple days.

## THE ANALYSIS

One clear warning with the Sirtfood Diet is its guarantee of large outcomes in a brief timeframe.

The manuscript has a major red sticker on the spread yelling that members will "lose 7 lbs. in 7 days." These kinds of cases regularly demonstrate diets looking to sucker individuals who are edgy to shed pounds, not diets planned for helping individuals make durable lifestyle changes. The "convenient solution" guarantee sets unreasonable desires for dieters, who may be persuaded they can keep on getting in shape at that emotional rate past multi week. Genuine, manageable weight loss is generally accomplished by shedding a couple of pounds seven days.

"I wouldn't be a major aficionado of supporting this kind of eating where it centers on losing a great deal of weight in a short measure of time," says enlisted dietitian Tavis Piattoly, who works as a sustenance advisor to the New Orleans Saints and New Orleans Pelicans. "A great deal of the weight will be water and potentially even muscle tissue."

Additionally, the calorie limitations during the principal week could be out and out risky, particularly if you're a competitor or dynamic individual. Competitors live exceptionally dynamic lifestyles, and young people need a greater number of calories than grown-ups significantly to help legitimate development. Albeit a calorie shortage is the way to getting thinner, too enormous a deficiency can cause issues like constant weariness and absence of core interest. NFL All-Pro guarded end J. J. Watt as of late felt the depleting impacts of a huge calorie shortfall and had to make some genuine diet changes to remain sharp.

Past the principal week, the center shifts from calorie-including to eating dinners high in sirtfoods. This is commonly a nice thought, since most of the nourishments associated with the Sirtfood Diet are profoundly nutritious. They're plant-based nourishments, low in calories and high in fiber, protein, nutrients, cancer prevention agents and phytochemicals. They're additionally substantially more difficult to gorge than profoundly handled nourishments.

Nonetheless, the entire "sirtuin activator" thing most likely assumes to a lesser extent a job in the intensity of sirtfoods than the remainder of their nourishing profile. Berries and kale is route preferred for you over treats and chips, whether or not they contain sirtuin activators. If you begin eating more plant-based nourishments, you're going to feel much improved—it's actually that basic.

## THE VERDICT

We praise the Sirtfood Diet for its emphasis on eating more plant-based nourishments; however it's unquestionably not an ideal diet.

The underlying calorie limitations are unreasonably exacting for some individuals, and the guarantee of seven pounds of weight loss in the initial seven days is anything but a solid methodology. The huge spotlight on sirtuins is likewise somewhat odd, since the exploration of sirtuins (and specifically, their job in weight the executives) is as yet starter. The sirtfoods remembered for the Sirtfood Diet are for the most part sound plant-based nourishments high in an assortment of supplements. We're speculating a great many different supplements and mixes in these nourishments (the majority of which are well-examined than sirtuin activators) are the genuine motivation behind why individuals are revealing sirtfoods assist them with feeling and look better. A lot of sound nourishments are excluded from the Sirtfood Diet and maintaining a strategic distance from them exclusively considering that it is absolutely superfluous.

If you're hoping to get more fit, your initial step ought to be to eliminate refined sugar items (pop, treats, and so on.) and excursions to the drive-through. Supplant those nourishments with plant-based alternatives and drink more water. If you're eating the correct sorts of nourishments, the amount you're eating shouldn't be a significant issue.

You should likewise meet with a wellbeing proficient or

enlisted dietitian. They can customize an arrangement for you as opposed to utilizing the "one-size-fits-all" approach numerous trend diets depend on. What's more, recollect—gradual advancement is often the most secure and the most manageable approach to getting more fit.

The Sirtfood Diet: the most recent in a not insignificant rundown of BS faddy diets customers, companions, and family, have sent me for my expert scrutinize. I figured that if they were asking, then others must have questions as well. This is a quite extensive manuscript so here's the TL: DR - this diet is false, don't get the manuscript, and work with a qualified nutritionist.

**Still with me? How about we separate it.**

Most importantly, we have to comprehend what sirtfoods are, and to get that, we have to realize what sirtuins are. You all prepared for a little science? Here we go. Sirtuins have been embroiled in keeping fat cells from copying, a wonder known as adipogenesis (fat cells being the Latin for fat) (lol jk, yet fat means fat).

Along these lines, the hypothesis is then, that specific nourishments can upregulate the declaration of the SIR qualities. Every one of that implies are those sure nourishments sending messages to our DNA to instruct them to make a greater amount of the sirtuin proteins. In this way, more sirtfoods=more sir proteins. Alright? It's somewhat more muddled than that, yet you get the thought.

The creators of TSD, made this a stride further and essentially arrived at the resolution that if you make a diet up of a lot of these alleged 'sirtfoods' you'll not just impact individuals' fat cells and make them free a lot of weight, yet they'll adequately get undying all the while.

The diet is separated into three phases as clarified here, yet to sum things up: The "Hyper Success Phase" (motivated naming their folks), whereby dieters are limited to 1000kcals every day made up of three sirtfood green juices and a sirtfood rich dinner. For three days in a row. Stage two then, gets an extra 500kcal, on the grounds that you dump one of the juices and supplant it with real nourishment – sirtfoods, however. Recollect that, it's significant. Toward the week's end you go into the support period of 3 sirtfood rich dinners in addition to a sirtfood juice.

The creators put this diet under a magnifying glass in their first class, private individuals rec center, where members (n=40) got instructional courses with a fitness coach and were under the creators' master healthful direction. They paid around £1,500 for the benefit as well. I think we'd all concur this was a thorough and replicable examination, no?

To be completely forthright: I have not perused the manuscript (hello, nobody sent me a development duplicate and nobody's paying me for composing this poo). Anyway, in view of what I can gather from the popular press (and yes I realize it would not stand up as an authentic source in the court of science, yet simply stay with me), here is every one of the issues I have with The Sirtfood Diet. An answer, if you will.

## 7 POUNDS IN 7 DAYS

In this way, the large case from TSD is that you can lose 7lbs in 7 days. Goggins and Matten guarantee that their diet isn't about weight loss; it's about wellbeing, and however these 7 out of 7 are key to their showcasing technique. It's spread all around the title page of the manuscript FFS. In addition to the fact that this is somewhat weight loss impractical, sensational, and unfortunate, it tends to be mentally harming to set somebody up with this sort of ridiculous desire for the diet. 1-2lbs every week is the suggestion for weight loss. It doesn't occur without any forethought, it's moderate and steady and hella baffling. My speculation is that it didn't all go on medium-term, so we have to have practical assumptions regarding losing it as well.

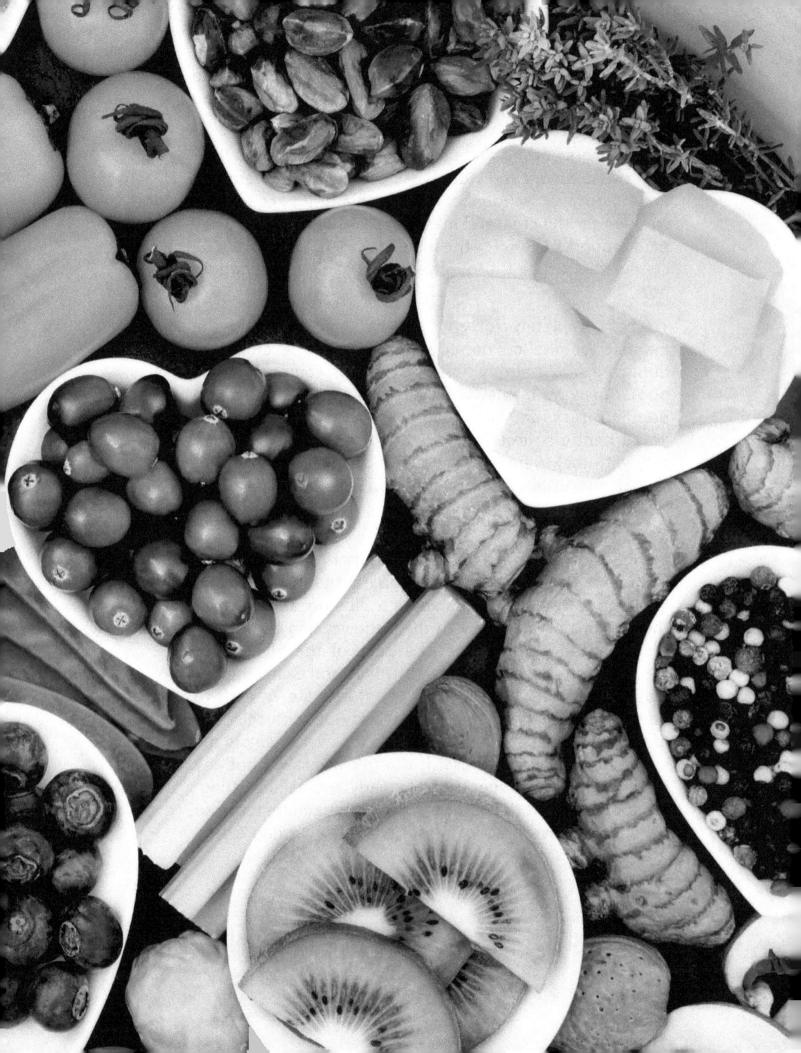

# CHAPTER 02

# How to Activate Your Skinny Gene without Fasting

The skinny gene-diet is not difficult to follow and is divided into two phases. The first phase lasts 7 days and is more restrictive and difficult, especially for the first 3 days.

From the fourth to the seventh day, instead, you can ingest 1,500 calories per day by taking three green juices and two solid meals composed of foods rich in sirtuins.

What makes the sirtfood diet different from the others is its "inclusion" philosophy. In fact, it is not based on the total or partial exclusion of some foods from your diet. Rather, it suggests which foods should be added to lose weight more easily. In this way, you will no longer have to undergo excessive deprivation or exhausting willpower. And you won't have to resort to expensive supplements or products with mysterious components. By eating a balanced diet and supporting it, if desired, with proper physical activity, according to the two nutritionists, you can lose about 3.5kg in a week. These genes are sirtuins.

They became famous thanks to an important study conducted in 2003, during which scientists analyzed a particular substance, resveratrol, present in the peel of black grapes, red wine, and yeast, which would produce the same effects of calorie restriction without need to decrease your daily calories intake. Researchers found that other substances in red wine had a similar effect, which would explain the benefits of consuming this drink and why those who consume it get less fat.

This naturally stimulated the search for other foods containing a high concentration of these nutrients, capable of producing such a beneficial effect on the body, and studies gradually discovered several.

After the discovery in 2003, the enthusiasm for the benefits of sort's food skyrocketed. Studies revealed that these foods don't just mimic the effects of calorie restriction. They also act as super regulators of the entire metabolism: they burn fat, increase muscle mass, and improve the health of our cells. The world of medical research was close to the most important nutritional discovery of the century. Unfortunately, a mistake was made. The sirtfood diet, however, does not share this pharmaceutical approach, which seeks (so far without result) to concentrate the benefits of these complex nutrients of plant origin into a single drug. Instead of waiting for the pharmaceutical industry to transform the nutrients of the foods we eat into a miraculous product (which may not work anyway), the sirtfood diet consists of eating these substances in their natural form that of food, to take full advantage of them. This is the basis of the pilot experiment of the sirtfood diet, with which the creators intended to create a diet containing the richest sources of sirt foods and observe their effects.

During their studies, Glen Matten and Aidan Goggins discovered that the best sirt foods are consumed regularly by populations who boast the lowest incidence of diseases and obesity in the world.

The Kuna Indians, in the American continent, seem immune from hypertension and with very low levels of obesity, diabetes, cancer, and early death thanks to the intake of cocoa, excellent sirt food. In Okinawa, Japan, sirt food, dry physique, and longevity go hand in hand. In India, the passion for spicy foods, especially turmeric, gives good results in the fight against cancer. And in the traditional Mediterranean diet, which the rest of the western world envies, obesity is contained, and chronic diseases are the exception, not the norm. extra virgin olive oil, wild green leafy vegetables, dried fruit, berries, red wine, dates, and aromatic herbs are all effective sirt foods, and they are all present in the Mediterranean diet. The scientific world has had to surrender to the evidence: it seems that the Mediterranean diet is more effective than reducing calories to lose weight and more effective than drugs to eliminate diseases.

Although sirt foods are not a mainstay of nutrition in most of the western world today, the situation was quite different in the past. They were a basic element, and if many have become rare and others have even disappeared, it is definitely possible to reverse the course of this.

The good news is that you don't have to be a top athlete, and not even sporty, to enjoy the same benefits. We took advantage of everything we learned about sirt foods thanks to the pilot study by kx and the work done with sportsmen, and we adapted it to create a diet suitable for anyone who wants to lose weight while improving health.

It is not necessary to practice unsustainable fasting or to undergo endless sessions in the gym (although, of course, practicing a little physical activity would be good for you). It is not an expensive diet, nor will it waste your time, and all the foods recommended in the diet are readily available. The only accessory you will need is an extractor or centrifuge. Unlike other diets, which tell you what to eliminate, this diet tells you what to eat.

Generally, you can eat foods that are high in protein and low in fat. Among the meat-based recipes, you can choose, for example, chicken with red onion and black cabbage, turkey with cauliflower couscous, turkey escalope with capers and parsley. For fish dishes, sautéed salmon fillet, sautéed prawns, or baked marinated cod are fine.

Recipes of side dishes, light and tasty, can be prepared with beans, lentils, aubergine cut into wedges, and cooked in the oven, Waldron salad, or red onions. And as for dessert, you can eat delicious and healthy strawberries, with a very high content of sirtuins. Plus, remember that 15-20g of dark chocolate are allowed every day.

The green juice is an important part of the diet, because

it has the ability to cleanse and detoxify, and will be the protagonist in the first week of the sirt prog.

Sirt foods are particularly rich in special nutrients of plant origin recently discovered, which, stimulated by fasting, activate the genes of thinness.

The foods suggested in the sirtfood diet are fresh, genuine and easily available, such as extra virgin olive oil, dark chocolate, citrus fruits, strawberries, apples, cabbage, celery, spinach, buckwheat, blueberries, nuts, soya beans, rocket salad, red onion, coffee, green tea**, red wine, chilli pepper***, tofu, turmeric, and dates.

In addition, combined with each other or with other foods, they allow you to create very tasty dishes.

# CHAPTER 03

# THE SCIENTIFIC BASIS OF SIRT DIET

And here is the note that, in general, represents the most painful point for those who develop a diet: the opinion of science. Overall, expert opinion on the Sirtfood diet is mixed. There is in-depth and unequivocal research that highlights the numerous benefits of some of the foods indicated. These include coffee, green tea, dark chocolate and green leafy vegetables. Many of these foods can also support healthy weight loss. However, it remains to be proven scientifically whether or not they promote weight loss by activating sirtuins. The weight loss resulting from the Sirtfood diet could be attributed to the consumption of fewer calories and more fiber, which occurs in different types of diets, even more varied. For example, a Mediterranean diet strengthened by so-called sirtfoods would already be a good plan to start losing a few pounds. Finally, let's not forget that it is always important to consult a doctor before starting a specific diet, whatever it is. Only in this way will it be possible to define a personalized scheme to measure one's nutritional needs and objectives. What is this diet based on? On the search for the so-called sirtuins. When called into question, a class of fundamental proteins is framed to maintain cellular health.

Some plant compounds, scientific data in hand, would be able to increase the levels of sirtuins in the body. Equally fundamental is to specify that scientific research on the benefits that the increase of sirtuins in the body can entail is still in the initial phase and with results that mainly concern animal models.

Interesting in this regard is a 2004 study, which involved a team from the Massachusetts Institute of Technology and which allowed to discover that, in a sample of mice, sirtuins can act on the genes that mediate the conservation of fat.

However, the scientists point out that even though the Sirt diet is characterized by the presence of a large number of healthy foods, the calorie restriction it recommends can prove difficult to sustain. In light of this, if you intend to undertake it, it is advisable to consult your doctor and be followed step by step. The benefits of this diet are different and science also agrees. One is the fact that the calorie limit is indicative and not a goal to be achieved. Another advantage is that the dishes on offer are very satisfying. This way you won't have the hunger attacks typical of other diets. The caloric restriction of the diet even in the most intensive phase is not drastic and Sirt foods have a satiating effect, which prevents us from going hungry at meals. The opinions, as always, are conflicting; people who claim to have benefited from this kind of diet and doctors and nutritionists who warn people from relying on alternative food regimes that promise to lose weight in a short time and without too much effort. Some nutritionists then pointed out that this diet is based on too weak scientific research and that people simply say they lose weight by following this diet because their theoretical calorie requirement would be much more than that taken into consideration by this diet.

Furthermore, some research has highlighted how sirtuin proteins play an important role in metabolism and fats, but this does not mean that by eating the foods offered by this diet people can lose weight. In short, for doctors, nutritionists and scientists, the opinions are conflicting and in some cases, they consider it another alternative diet that is mixed with the many food regimes that promise to lose weight in a short time.

There are essentially three criticisms made by scientists and nutritionists about this diet:

    1. It is true that Sirt makes you lose weight, but this

would depend on the fact that the foods included in the menu are low in fat and calories. That Sirt foods can also regulate metabolism has so far been proven only in animal studies.

2. The only scientific research supporting this theory is the pilot study mentioned in the manuscript by Matten and Goggins: it was conducted by nutritionists themselves in a London gym on a limited sample (39 people) followed only for 7 days. So the results (-3.2 kg on average) are difficult to generalize. Sirtfood foods are rich in beneficial properties, but the 3 weeks of the Sirt diet, restrictive and low-calorie, are a hit and run remedy difficult to carry out and potentially risky if prolonged over time.

3. Although the Sirtfoods diet includes many healthy foods, rich in fiber, vitamins and antioxidant elements also present in the Mediterranean Diet, it is not entirely free of side effects.

In fact, it is a low-calorie diet (1000-1500 calories) that focuses mainly on fruit, vegetables, herbs and spices. But it is also true that fish, white meat and carbohydrates also appear on the menu, but if the diet is not customized, it is possible to run into nutritional deficiencies (e.g. iron, proteins, calcium and sugar), tiredness, fatigue, sudden changes in mood, excessive weight loss, headache, difficulty concentrating, halitosis and pressure drops.

Also, drinking vegetable concentrates every day for three weeks could alter your metabolism and cause nausea and intestinal discomfort. What could make this diet dangerous would be the belief that you can sustain this type of nutrition for long periods. But if you follow the recommendations of the creators of the diet, this risk does not exist.

However, experts note that the Sirt diet is not suitable for children and adolescents, people who are underweight, wasting or recovering, and in the presence of nutritional deficiencies or eating disorders. In addition, it should only be followed on the advice and medical supervision of pregnant or breastfeeding women, elderly people and menopausal ladies, and in case of diabetes, metabolic diseases, liver and kidney problems, gastrointestinal disorders and chronic conditions.

In any case, it should be remembered that this diet should not always be followed: for some people it will be necessary to repeat it only twice a year, while for others once every three months. This depends on the build, the metabolism and many factors that vary in each of us.

# Chapter 04

# The Top 20 Sirt Food and Other Ingredient for a Sirt-Full Diet

Sirtfoods are plant foods that are rich in specific polyphenols that activate our sirtuin genes. Eating these sirtfoods turns on a process of recycling in our cells to clear up all the clutter and waste that grows up with age and normally causes ill health. Our cells tap into our fat stores to fuel that recycling process. It resulted in rejuvenated cells, a lack of fitness, strength and weight.

Sirtfoods are the innovative way our sirtuin genes can be regulated in the best way possible. These are particularly rich wonder foods in unique natural plant chemicals, called polyphenols, which have the ability to activate our sirtuin genes by clicking on them. Essentially, they emulate the results of fasting and exercise and thus offer impressive benefits by helping the body better regulate blood sugar levels, burning fat, building muscle, and improving wellbeing and memory.

Because they are stationary, plants have developed a highly sophisticated system of stress-response and produce polyphenols to help them adapt to their environment's challenges. When we eat these plants, we benefit from consuming the polyphenol these nutrients. They have a profound effect: they activate our own innate pathways of stress-response.

While all plants have stress-response systems, only some have evolved to produce remarkable amounts of polyphenols that activate sirtuin. These are sirt-foods. Their finding means that there is now a revolutionary new way to trigger the sirtuin genes, instead of rigid fasting regimens or arduous exercise programs: consuming an ample diet of sirtfoods. Most of all, the diet involves putting food (sirt) on your plate, and not getting it off.

**1. Capers**

**2. Arugula**

**3. Celery**

**4. Chilies**

**5. Cocoa**

**6. Coffee**

**7. Extra Virgin Olive Oil**

**8. Garlic**

**9. Green Tea (especially Match)**

**10. Kale**

**11. Medjool Dates**

**12. Parsley**; It is a gastronomic conundrum. It so often appears in recipes, yet so often it's the green token man. At best, we serve a couple of chopped sprigs and tossed as an afterthought on a meal, at worst a solitary sprig for decorative purposes only. Either way, there on the plate, it is often still languishing long after we've eaten finish. This culinary style derives from its common use in ancient Rome as a garnish for eating after meals in order to restore oxygen, rather than being part of the meal itself. And what a shame, because parsley is a fantastic food that packs a vivid and refreshing flavor that is a character filled with.

**13. Red Endive**

**14. Red Onions**; Red Onions have been a dietary staple, being one of the first crops to be grown, around 5,000 years ago. With such a long history of use and such strong health-giving properties, many cultures that came before us have revered onions.

**15. Red Wine**

**16. Soy**; Soy products have a long history as an important part of the diet of many countries in Asia-Paci, such as China, Japan, and Korea. After observing that high soy-consuming countries had significantly lower levels of certain cancers, particularly breast and prostate, researchers first turned on to soy.

**17. Strawberries**; Strawberries Fruit has been increasingly vilified, getting a bad rap in the rising fervor against sugar. Luckily, such a malignant image couldn't be more undeserved for berry-lovers. While all the berries are powerhouses of nutrition, strawberries gain their top twenty Sirtfood status due to their sirtuin activator set in abundance.

**18. Turmeric**; Turmeric, a cousin of ginger, is the latest kid in food trends on the block with Google calling it the 2015 ingredient "breakout star." While we are only turning to it nowhere in the West, it has been valued for thousands of years in Asia, for both culinary and medical reasons. Incredibly, India is generating almost the entire world's turmeric supply, eating 80 percent of it itself. Along with the "golden spice" benefits we saw on pages 60-61, in Asia, turmeric is used to treat skin disorders such as acne, psoriasis, dermatitis, and rash. Before Indian weddings, there is a ritual where the turmeric paste is applied as a skin beauty treatment to the bride and groom but also to symbolize the warding off evil.

**19. Walnuts**; Walnuts lead the way as the number one nut for health, according to the NuVal system, which ranks foods according to how safe they are and has been endorsed by the American College of Preventive Medicine. But what really makes walnuts stand out for us is how they stand out against conventional thinking: they are high in fat and calories, yet well-established for weight reduction and the risk of metabolic diseases such as cardiovascular disease and diabetes being reduced. That is the strength of triggering the sirtuin.

20. Buckwheat

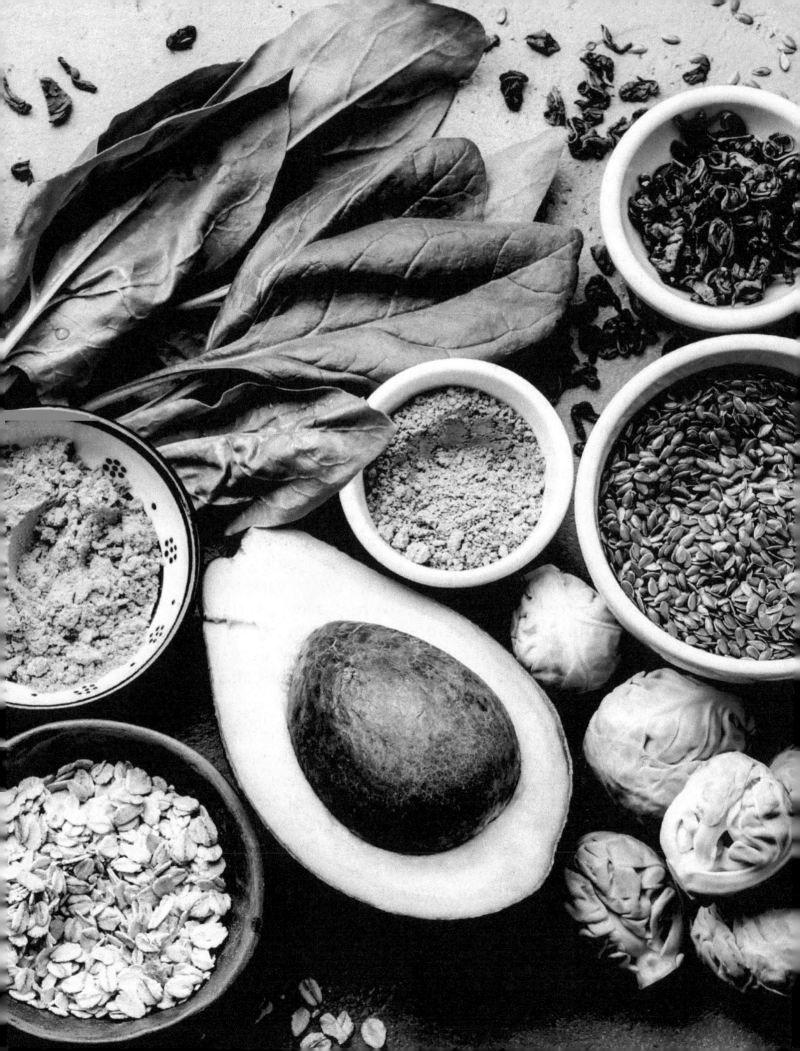

# CHAPTER 05

# Diet Sirt and Physical Exercise

## JOINING EXERCISE WITH THE SIRTFOOD DIET SIRTFOOD DIET AND EXERCISE

With 52% of Americans admitting that they think that its simpler to do their charges than to see how to eat steadily, it's fundamental to present a type of eating that turns into a lifestyle as opposed to a coincidental prevailing fashion diet. For a few of us it may not be that difficult to get thinner or hold a solid weight, however the Sirtfood diet can help the individuals who are battling. Be that as it may, shouldn't something be said about joining the Sirtfood diet with work out, is it fitting to stay away from practice totally or present it once you have begun the diet?

## THE SIRT DIET PRINCIPLES

With an expected 650 million hefty grown-ups internationally, it's critical to discover smart dieting and exercise systems that are feasible, don't deny you of all that you appreciate, and don't expect you to practice all week. The Sirtfood diet does only that. The thought is that sure nourishments will dynamic the 'thin quality' pathways which are normally actuated by fasting and exercise. Fortunately certain nourishment and drink, including dull chocolate and red wine, contain synthetic substances called polyphenols that enact the qualities that copy the impacts of activity and fasting.

## EXERCISE DURING THE INITIAL BARELY ANY WEEKS

During the main week or two of the diet where your calorie admission is diminished, it is reasonable to stop or lessen practice while your body adjusts to fewer calories. Tune in to your body and if you feel exhausted or have less vitality than expected, don't work out. Rather guarantee that you stay concentrated on the rules that apply to a solid lifestyle, for example, including satisfactory day by day levels of fiber, protein and products of the soil.

## WHEN THE DIET TURNS INTO A LIFESTYLE

When you do practice it's critical to devour protein in a perfect world an hour after your workout. Protein fixes muscles after exercise, lessens irritation and can help recuperation. There are an assortment of plans which incorporate protein which will be ideal for post-practice utilization, for example, the sirt stew con carne or the turmeric chicken and kale serving of mixed greens. If you need something lighter you could attempt the sirt blueberry smoothie and include some protein powder for included advantage. The kind of wellness you do will be down to you, however workouts at home will permit you to pick when to work out, and the sorts of activities that suit you and are short and helpful.

The Sirtfood diet is an incredible approach to change your dietary patterns, shed pounds and feel more advantageous. The underlying not many weeks may challenge you yet it's imperative to check which nourishments are ideal to eat and which scrumptious plans suit you. Be benevolent to yourself in the initial barely any weeks while your body adjusts and takes practice simple if you decide to do it by any stretch of the imagination. If you are as of now somebody who moderates or extreme exercise then it might be that you can carry on as ordinary, or deal with your wellness as per the adjustment in diet. Similarly as with any diet and exercise changes, it's about the individual and how far you can propel yourself.

Minerals and nutrients for which ladies may require supplements incorporate calcium, iron, Vitamins B6, B12 and D. Men, be that as it may, need to focus on fiber, magnesium, Vitamins B9, C and E.

That reason applies to weight loss diets also. People's nourishment necessities sway in which weight loss diets are increasingly compelling for each sex.

If you're similar to the vast majority, you've seen an astounding number of weight loss projects and patterns go back and forth; practically every one of them has their benefits and practically every one of them work — incidentally. Weight the executives and therapeutic experts fight collectively that the deep rooted, proven blend of good sustenance and ordinary exercise is the most ideal approach to adequately shed pounds and keep it off.

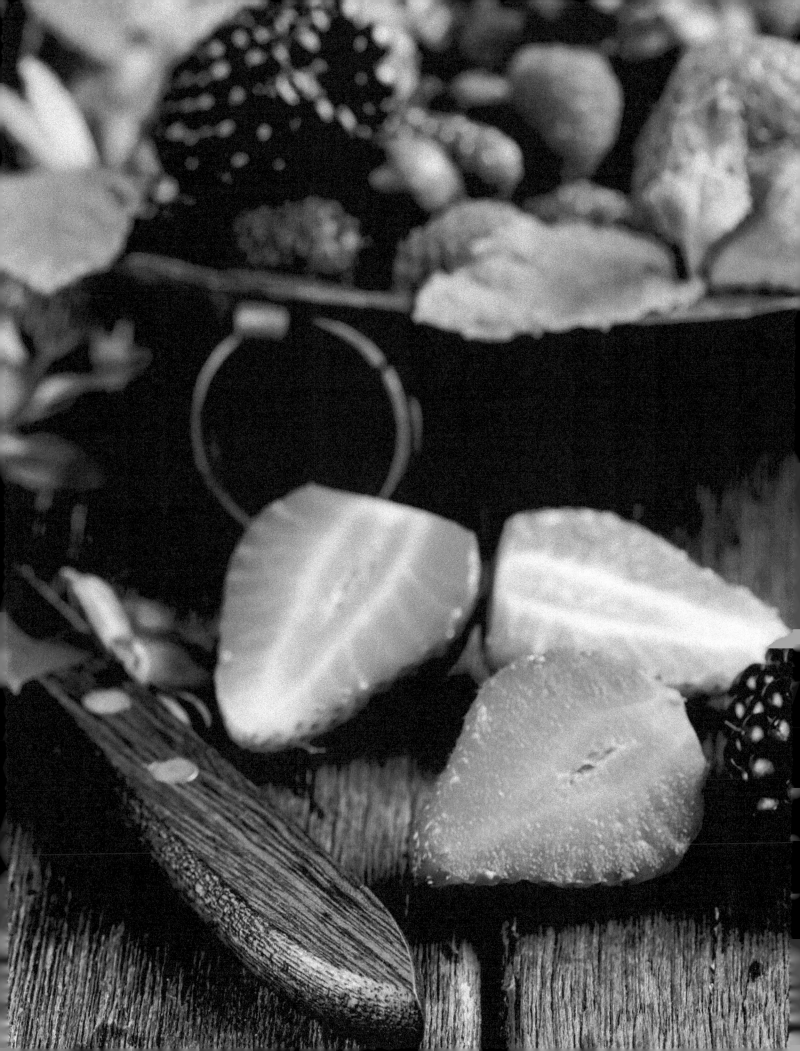

# Chapter 06

# Sirtfoods in Detail

The basis of the sirtuin diet can be explained in simple terms or in complex ways. It is important to understand how and why it works however, so that you can appreciate the value of what you are doing. It is important to also know why these sirtuin rich foods help to help you maintain fidelity to your diet plan. Otherwise, you may throw something in your meal with less nutrition that would defeat the purpose of planning for one rich in sirtuins. Most importantly, this is not a dietary fad, and as you will see, there is much wisdom contained in how humans have used natural foods even for medicinal purposes, over thousands of years.

To understand how the Sirtfood diet works, and why these particular foods are necessary, we will look at the role they play in the human body.

Sirtuin activity was first researched in yeast, where a mutation caused an extension in the yeast's lifespan. Sirtuins were also shown to slow aging in laboratory mice, fruit flies, and nematodes. As research on Sirtuins proved to transfer to mammals, they were examined for their use in diet and slowing the aging process. The sirtuins in humans are different in the typing but they essentially work in the same ways and reasons.

There are seven "members" that make up the sirtuin family. It is believed that sirtuins play a big role in regulating certain functions of cells including proliferation (reproduction and growth of cells), apoptosis (death of cells). They promote survival and resist stress to increase longevity.

They are also seen to block neurodegeneration (loss of function of the nerve cells in the brain). They conduct their housekeeping functions by cleaning out toxic proteins and supporting the brain's ability to change and adapt to different conditions, or to recuperate (i.e., brain plasticity). As part of this they also help reduce chronic inflammation, and reduce something called oxidative stress. Oxidative stress is when there are too many cell-damaging free radicals circulating in the body, and the body cannot catch up by combating them with anti-oxidants. These factors are related to age-related illness and weight as well, which again, brings us back to a discussion of how they actually work.

You will see labels in Sirtuins that start with "SIR," which represents "Silence Information Regulator" genes. They do exactly that, silence or regulate, as part of their functions. The seven sirtuins that humans work with are: SIRT1, SIRT2, SIRT3, SIRT4, SIRT 5, SIRT6 and SIRT7. Each of these types is responsible for different areas of protecting cells. They work by either stimulating or turning on certain gene expressions, or by reducing and turning off other gene expressions. This essentially means that they can influence genes to do more or less of something, most of which they are already programmed to do.

Through enzyme reactions, each of the SIRT types affects different areas of cells that are responsible for the metabolic processes that help to maintain life. This is also related to what organs and functions they will affect.

For example, the SIRT6 causes an expression of genes in humans that affect skeletal muscle, fat tissue, brain, and heart. SIRT 3 would cause an expression of genes that affect the kidneys, liver, brain and heart.

If we tie these concepts together, you can see that the Sirtuin proteins can change the expression of genes, and in the case of the Sirtfood diet we care about how sirtuins can turn off those genes that are responsible for speeding up aging and for weight management.

The other aspect to this conversation of sirtuins is the function and the power of calorie restriction on the human body. Calorie restriction is simply eating fewer calories. This coupled with exercise and reducing stress is usually a combination of weight loss. Calorie restriction has also proven across much research in animals and humans to increase one's lifespan.

We can look further at the role of sirtuins with calorie restriction, and using the SIRT3 protein which has a role in metabolism and aging. Amongst all of the effects of the protein on gene expression, (such as preventing cells from dying, reducing tumors from growing, etc.), we want to understand the effects of SIRT3 on weight for the purpose of this manuscript.

The SIRT3 has high expression in those metabolically active tissues as we stated earlier, and its ability to express itself increases with caloric restriction, fasting, and exercise. On the contrary, it will express itself less when the body has a high fat, high calorie-riddled diet.

The last few highlights of sirtuins are their role in regulating telomeres and reducing inflammation which also helps with staving off disease and aging.

Telomeres are sequences of proteins at the ends of chromosomes. When cells divide these get shorter. As we age they get shorter and other stressors to the body also will contribute to this. Maintaining these longer telomeres is the key to slower aging. In addition, proper diet, along with exercise and other variables can lengthen telomeres. SIRT6 is one of the sirtuins that, if activated, can help with DNA damage, inflammation and oxidative stress. SIRT1 also helps with inflammatory response cycles that are related to many age-related diseases.

Calories restriction, as we mentioned earlier, can extend life to some degree.

Since this, as well as fasting, is a stressor, these factors will stimulate the SIRT3 proteins to kick in and protect the body from the stressors and excess free radicals. Again, the telomere length is affected as well.

To sum up, all of this information also shows that, contrary to some people's beliefs that in terms of genetics, such as "it is what it is" or "it is my fate because Uncle Joe has something..." through our own lifestyle choices, and what we are exposed to, we can influence action and changes in our genes. This is quite an empowering thought, and yet another reason why you should be excited to have a science-based diet such as the Sirtfood diet, available to you.

Having laid this all out before you, you should be able to appreciate how and why these miraculous compounds work in your favor, to keep you youthful, healthy, and lean If they are working hard for you, don't you feel that you should do something too?

# FOOD PLAN ON THE FIRST 7 DAYS

| Days | Breakfast | Lunch | Dinner | Snack |
|---|---|---|---|---|
| Day 01 | Sirtfood Pears N' Spinach Juice | Sirtfood Persimmon - Mint Magic Juice | Sirtfood Steak Diane | Sirtfood Minty Green Juice |
| Day 02 | Sirtfood Minty Green Juice | Sirtfood Protein Green Juice | Fried Rice Pineapple | Sirtfood Sunflower Spinach Juice |
| Day 03 | Sirtfood Persimmon-Mint Magic | Sirtfood Sunflower Spinach Juice | Garlic Anchovy Linguine | Sirtfood Pears N' Spinach Juice |
| Day 04 | Sirtfood Protein Green Juice | Sirtfood Persimmon - Mint Magic Juice | Sirtfood Fried Chicken | Sirtfood Cheddar Crackers |
| Day 05 | Sirtfood Sunflower Spinach Juice | Pinto Bean Spread | Taco Bell Spicy Tostada | Sirtfood Minty Green Juice |
| Day 06 | Sirtfood Persimmon - Mint Magic Juice | Sirtfood Protein Green Juice | Farfalle with Capers | Fluffy Orange Gelatin Pie |
| Day 07 | Sirtfood Pears N' Spinach Juice | Sirtfood Oriental Barbecued Pork | Sirtfood Artichoke And Egg Spread | Sirtfood Persimmon - Mint Magic Juice |

# CHAPTER 07

# Maintaining

Having seen these sometimes-incredible changes ourselves, we realize how much you're going to want to see much better results, not just retain all those advantages. Sirtfoods are, after all, designed to eat for life. The problem is how you adapt what you learned in Phase 1 into your regular dietary practice. That is precisely what inspired us to develop a fourteen-day maintenance plan designed to help you make the transition from Phase 1 to your more usual dietary regimen, thus helping to maintain and expand the benefits of the Sirtfood Diet further.

## WHAT TO EXPECT

You should maintain the weight loss results through Phase 2 and continue to lose weight gradually. Also, the one striking thing we've seen with the Sirtfood Diet is that most or all of the weight people lose is from fat and that many put some muscle on. So, we would like to warn you again not to measure your success solely based on the numbers. Look in the mirror to see if you look leaner and more toned, see how well your clothes fit and lap up the compliments you'll get from others.

Note that just as weight loss occurs, the health benefits will increase. In implementing the fourteen-day maintenance plan, you are helping to lay the foundations for a lifelong health future.

## HOW TO FOLLOW PHASE 2

The key to success in this process is having your diet packed full of Sirtfoods. We've put together a seven-day meal schedule for you to adapt to make it as easy as possible, with tasty family-friendly meals, filled with Sirtfoods every day to the rafters. Now what you need to do is to implement Seven Day Program twice to fulfill Phase 2's fourteen days.

On each of fourteen days, your diet will consist of:

Three times balanced sirtfood meals

1-time sirtfood green juice

1 - 2 times optional sirtfood snacks

Also, when you have to eat those, there are no strict laws. Be agile throughout every day and suit them. Two basic thumb-rules are:

Take sirtfood green juice either in the morning or at least half an hour before breakfast.

Try your best to take dinner by 7 PM.

## PORTION SIZES

In Phase 2, our attention is not on calorie counting. For the average person, this is not a practical approach or even a good one over the long term. Instead, we concentrate on healthy servings, really well-balanced meals, and most notably, filling up on Sirtfoods so that you can continue to benefit from their fat-burning and health-promoting impact.

We've even designed the meals in the plan to make them satiate, making you stay full for longer. This coupled with Sirtfoods' innate appetite-regulating power, ensures you're not going to spend the following 14 days feeling thirsty, but rather comfortably fulfilled, well-fed, and highly well-nourished.

Just like in Phase 1, try to listen and be driven by your appetite. When you prepare meals according to our guidelines and notice that you are easily full before you finish a meal, then stop eating is perfectly fine!

## WHAT TO DRINK

During Phase 2 you'll need to include one green juice every day. This is to keep you top with high Sirtfoods prices.

Just like in Phase 1, you will easily absorb other fluids in Phase 2. Our preferred beverages contain remaining plain water, bottled flavored water, coffee, and green tea. Whether black or white tea is your preference, feel free to enjoy it. The same goes for herbal teas. The best news is that during Phase 2, you will enjoy the occasional bottle of red wine. Due to its content of sirtuin-activating polyphenols, particularly resveratrol and piceatannol, red wine is a sirtfood that makes it the best choice of alcoholic beverage. However, with alcohol itself causing adverse effects on our fat cells, restraint is still safest, so we suggest restricting the drink to one glass of red wine with a meal for two to three days a week in Phase 2.

## RETURNING TO THREE MEALS

You enjoyed only one or two meals per day during Phase 1 and allowed you plenty of versatility when you eat your meals. As we are now back to a more normal routine and the well-tested practice of three meals a day, learning about breakfast is a good time.

Eating a good breakfast sets, us on for the day, raising our levels of energy and focus. Eating early holds our blood sugar and fat rates in balance, in terms of our metabolism. Breakfast is a good thing that is pointed out by a number of studies, usually showing that people who eat breakfast often are less prone to overweight.

The explanation for this is because of our internal clocks inside. Our bodies are asking us to feed early in expectation of when we will be most busy and need food. Yet, as many as a third of us will miss breakfasts on any given day. It's a classic symptom in our crazy modern life, and the feeling is there's simply not enough time to eat properly. But as you will see, with the nifty breakfasts we have laid out for you here, nothing could be further from the truth. Whether it's the Sirtfood smoothie that can be drunk on the go, the premade Sirt muesli, or the quick and easy Sirtfood scrambled eggs/tofu, finding those extra few minutes in the morning will reap dividends not only for your day but for your longer-term weight and health.

With Sirtfoods functioning to overcharge our energy levels, there's, even more, to learn from getting a hit from them early in the morning to continue your day. This is done not only by consuming a Sirtfood-rich meal but above all by including the green juice, which we suggest you have either first thing in the morning — at least thirty minutes before breakfast— or mid-morning. We get a lot of reports from our personal experience of people who first consume their green juice and don't feel hungry for a few hours afterward. If this is the impact it's having on you, taking a couple of hours until having breakfast is perfectly fine. Just don't miss this one. Instead, with a good breakfast, you should kick off your day, and then wait two to three hours to have the green juice. Be versatile, and just go with anything that suits you.

## SIRTFOOD SNACKS

You should keep it when it comes to snacking or quit it. There is a long debate on whether consuming regular, smaller meals is better for weight loss, or just keeping to three balanced meals a day. The fact is that it does not matter.

The way we've designed the maintenance menu for you means you're going to eat three well-balanced Sirtfood-rich meals a day, and you may notice that you don't need a snack. But maybe you've been busy with the kids in the classroom, working out or dashing about and need something to take you into the following meal. And if that "little something" is going to give you a whammy of Sirtfood nutrients and taste delicious, then it's happy days. This is why we created our "Sirtfood bites." These smart little snacks are a genuinely guilt-free treat made entirely from Sirtfoods: dates, walnuts, cocoa, extra virgin olive oil, and turmeric. We recommend eating one, or a maximum of two, per day for the days when you require them.

## SIRTIFYING YOUR MEAL

We saw that the only consistent diets are those of participation, not exclusion. Yet real success goes beyond this— the diet has to be consistent with living in modern days. Whether it's the ease of meeting the demands of our hectic lives or fitting in with our position at dinner parties as to the bon vivant, the way we eat should be trouble-free. You will appreciate your svelte body and beautiful smile, rather than thinking about the demands and limitations of kooky products.

What makes Sirtfoods so great is that they are available, common, and simple to include in your diet. Below, when you bridge the gap between step 1 and daily feeding, you can lay the foundations for a modern, better lifelong eating strategy.

The key principle is what we term the meals "Sirtifying." This is where we take popular meals, including many traditional classics, and we retain all the great taste with some smart modifications and easy Sirtfood inclusions but attach a lot of goodness to that. You'll see just how quickly this is done in Phase 2.

Highlights include our tasty smoothie Sirtfood for the ultimate on-the-go breakfast in a time-consuming environment and the easy turn from wheat to buckwheat to add extra flavor and zip to the much-loved pasta comfort food. While classic, famous dishes such as chili con carne and curry don't even need much improvement, with Sirtfood bonanzas providing traditional recipes. Yet who has said that fast food means bad health? If you prepare something yourself, we mix the true vivid tastes of a pizza and through the shame. There's no need to say goodbye to indulgence yet, as our smothered pancakes with berries and dark chocolate sauce have demonstrated. It's not even a treat, it's breakfast, and for you it's perfect. Simple changes: you keep eating the things that you enjoy when maintaining healthy weight and well-being. And that is Sirtfoods, the culinary movement.

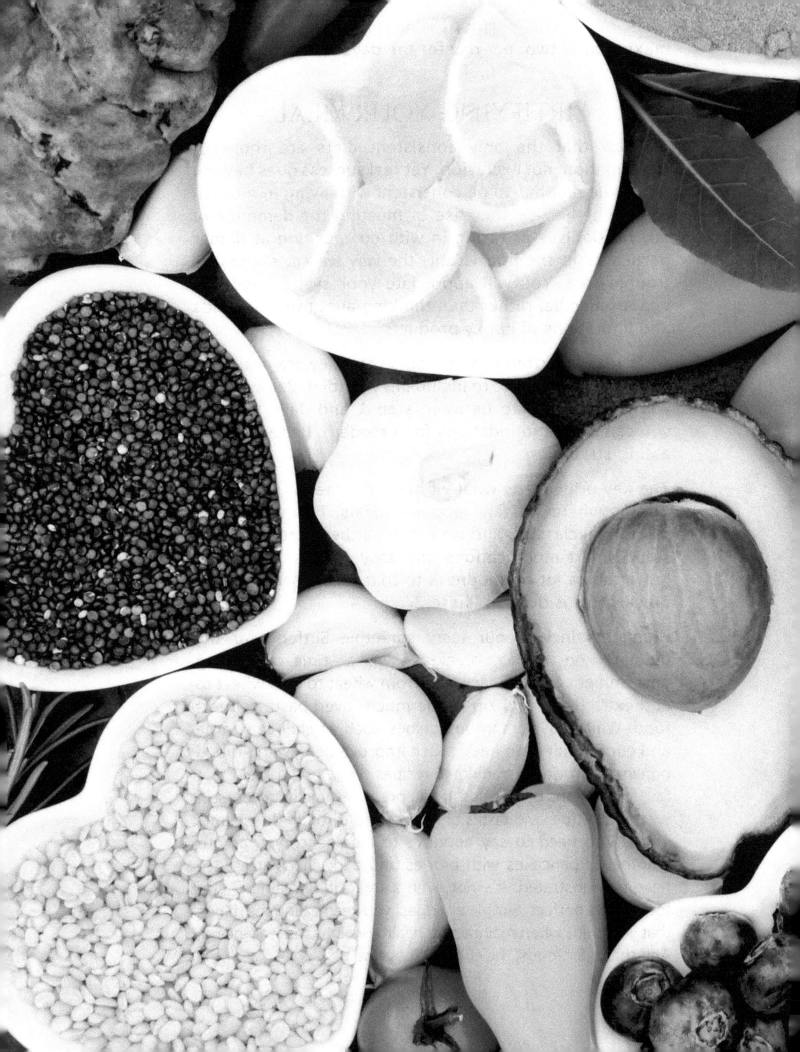

# Chapter 08

# Shopping List

All these would be the highest-rated foods to get a Sirtfood-rich diet program and ways to incorporate them into your everyday meals.

- **Carrots**
- **Celery**
- **Oil**
- **Pork loin**
- **All-purpose flour**
- **Apple cider**
- **Avocado**
- **Ground cumin**
- **Black pepper**
- **Salt**
- **Chicken**
- **Turkey Breasts**
- **Fish**
- **Yeast**
- **Kale**
- **Pineapple**
- **Mushrooms**
- **Tamari**

- **Dried thyme**
- **Smoked paprika**
- **Dry mustard**
- **Earth's - eye chilli.** Additionally sold as Thai chillies, they truly are stronger than ordinary chillies and packed with more nutritional elements. Utilize them to increase sour or sweet recipes.
- **Capers.**
- **Celery.** The leaves and hearts would be the most healthful part, and thus do not throw them off if you are mixing a shake-up.
- **Chicory.** Red is most beneficial but yellowish works too. Include it into a salad.
- **Cocoa.** The flavonol-rich type enhances blood pressure, blood glucose cholesterol and control. Search to get a high proportion of cacao.
- **Coffee.** Drink it shameful -- there are some signs that milk can lower the absorption of sirtuin-activating nutritional elements.
- **Extra virgin steak oil.** The extra-virgin type includes more sirt benefits, and also a far more pleasing, flavor.
- **Green tea or Matcha.** Add a piece of lemon juice to raise the absorption of sirtuin-producing nutritional elements. Matcha is much better, but really go Japanese, not Chinese, in order to steer clear of potential lead contamination.
- **Kale.** Includes huge levels of sirtuin-activating nutrition Quercentin and kaempferol. Scrub it with coconut oil and lemon juice and serve it as a salad.
- **Lovage.** It is an herb. Grow your personal onto a window sill and throw it in to stir fries.
- **Medjool dates.** They truly are a hefty 66 percent glucose, however in moderation -- do not raise glucose levels, also have been connected to reduced levels of diabetes and cardiovascular disease.

- **Parsley.** More than only a garnish -- it's saturated in apigenin. Throw into a juice or smoothie for the complete benefit. Chicory red is most beneficial, but yellowish functions fine. Throw it in a salad.

- **Red onion.** The reddish variety is healthier personally, and also sweet enough to eat raw. Stir it and put in to a salad or eat it with a hamburger.

- **Red wine.**

- **Rocket.**

- **Soy.**

- **Strawberries.**

- **Turmeric.** Evidence suggests the curcumin inside is anti-cancer properties. It's difficult for your human body to assimilate alone, however cooking it into fluid and including black pepper increases absorption.

- **Walnuts.** Full of calories and fat, but well recognized in lessening metabolic disorder. Mash them up with skillet to get a sirt-flavored pesto.

Sirtfoods are the revolutionary way of triggering our sirtuin genes in the finest way possible. All these are the miracle foods mainly full of specific all-natural plant compounds, called polyphenols that possess the capability to trigger our sirtuin genes by changing them. Essentially, they mimic the results of exercise and fasting; also doing this brings notable benefits by helping the system to better control glucose levels and burn fat, and build muscle and promote memory and health.

Because they're stationary plants also have developed an extremely complex stress-response system and also produce antioxidants to help them conform to the challenges in their own environment. Once we consume these plants, we additionally eat up this polyphenol nourishment. Their effect is deep: they trigger our very own inborn stress-response pathways.

Even though all plants possess stress-response techniques, just certain ones have grown to create impressive levels of sirtuin-activating polyphenols.

Would you eat meat about your Sirtfood diet?

The answer can be a resounding, yes. The diet not just comprises ingesting a healthful part of beef, it urges that protein become a crucial addition within a Sirtfood-based diet plan to reap the most benefit in maintaining metabolic process and lessening the muscle imbalance common in many fat loss programs

Leucine is an amino acid found in protein that divides and actually enriches the action of Sirtfoods, which usually means that the perfect solution to consume Sirtfoods is by simply mixing them with a chicken, beef or alternative supply of leucine like eggs or fish.

Poultry could be eaten (since it's a great source of protein, b vitamins, potassium and phosphorous), also that red-meat (still another superb source of iron, protein, calcium and vitamin b 12) might be consumed to 3 occasions (750g raw weight) weekly.

Foods saturated in Sirtuins (proteins which regulate cellular and metabolic purpose), can play a part in increasing our wellbeing, reducing inflammation, and also potentially helping in weight loss too. In the event you are worried this diet will soon be miserably restrictive, you are in fortune: those sirtuin-activating foods aren't simply full of good, for you polyphenols, but they're also diverse, flavorful, also might be incorporated to your own diet in many of creative methods.

The 1st sirtuin activator understood -- but the most effective known -- has been resveratrol, found in the skin of red grapes (and that's the reason why red wine is traditionally believed to continue to keep you healthy), pomegranates and Japanese knotweed.

Additional sirtuin activators soon followed, like catechins (seen in green tea extract and also presumed to work with cancer cells) and epicatechins in cocoa powder (accountable for its health benefits of chocolates).

However, research took away once the pharmaceutical giant GlaxoSmithKline bought the rights to generate artificial variations of resveratrol for 462 million. It hastens trailed such as a cancer treatment however, the consequences weren't impressive. This season the organization announced it had ceased the research.

However, it today seems eating Sirtfoods naturally full of sirtuin activators could be described as a much healthier, far better -- and cheaper -- alternative for supplements. It was considering the newest trials of Sirtfoods as well as also the Sirtfood dietary plan. Present results imply that Sirtfoods target precisely the exact same path for reducing weight and staying fit since dietary restriction and physical exercise. Red wine fans have a new cause to observe.

Even though analysing the results of resveratrol from the diet rhesus monkeys," dr. J.p. Hyatt, an associate professor at Georgetown university, along with his group of investigators found a resveratrol supplement that could counteract the bad effect of a superior fat/high sugar diet onto the thoracic muscles. In former animal studies, resveratrol has shown to improve the life span of mice and slow down the onset of cardiovascular disease. In 1 study, it revealed the results of aerobic exercise mice, which have been fed with a superior fat/high sugar free diet plan.

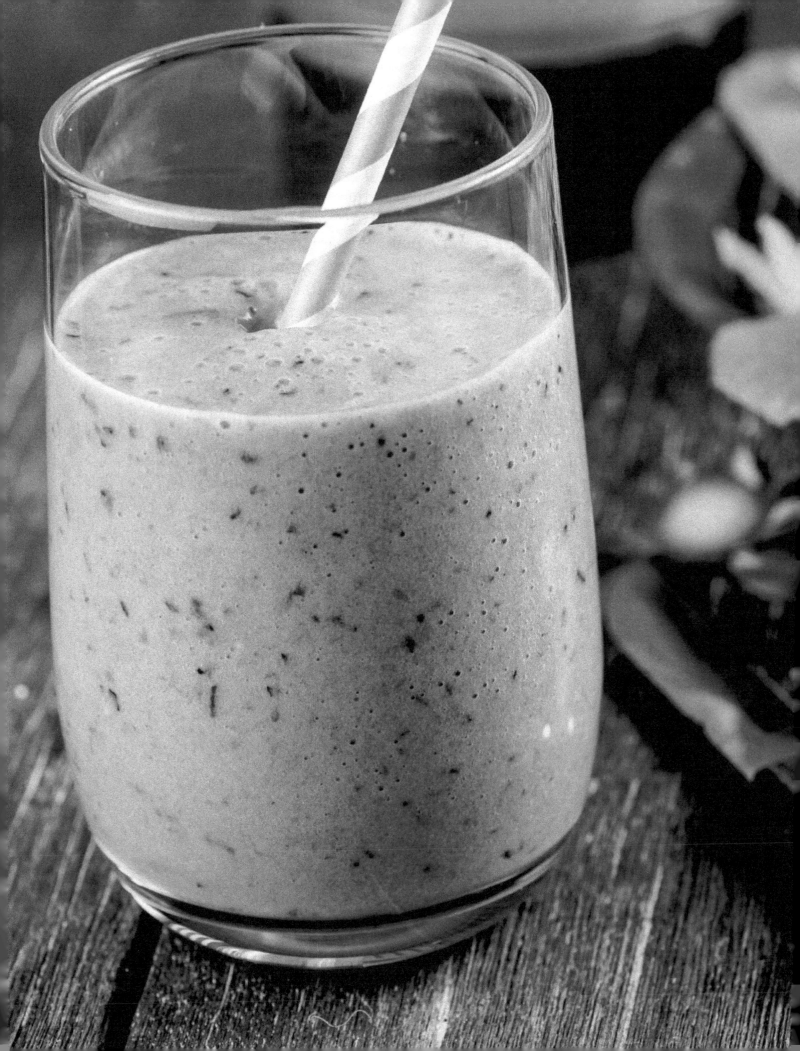

# Chapter 09

# The Sirtfood Green Juices and Smoothies

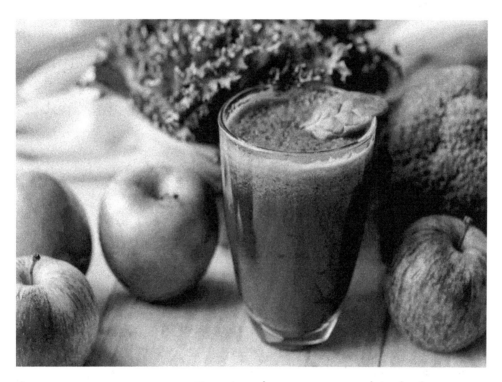

A very common question is: does a smoothie help you to lose weight? And the answer is yes! It can be a powerful and fantastic tool, but only when you know how to use it correctly.

Green juice and smoothies are a salvation for fading beauty. They help our body to fully detox for weight loss. And it's not only a delicious drink but it's also rich in nutrients that rejuvenate the skin, slow down the aging process and make your hair healthy and shiny again.

The following questions will you help decide if you should consider this type of diet:

- Don't think about your weight, pay attention to your body fat percentage - is it normal?
- Do you feel tired, even after you had a good rest?
- Do you suddenly crave something sweet during the day?
- Do you dull-looking hair and nails?
- Have you already tried a lot of diets without good results?

Even one "yes" is enough to think about your health and think about a detox cleanse diet. If you are determined to change your life with green smoothies, then here are some steps to follow for a successful start and the best results:

## NO MORE EXCESS BODY FAT AND CHRONIC DISEASES

What green juices and smoothies can help your body do is to get rid of excess fat, making your life much better without it. Its nutrients are responsible for regulating blood insulin levels in your body. When blood insulin's concentration is higher than normal, more fat is stored inside the body. It can increase the risks of dangerous diseases as renal impairment, heart disease, diabetes, and even several types of cancer, among others. That's why you should control your amount of visceral body fat.

## LIMIT THE TOXIC EXPOSURE ON YOUR BODY

Green juice and smoothies are a great source of natural nutrients that will make your body and immune system much stronger and reduce the inflammatory process. As the source of essential elements for our body, a green smoothie includes natural sugars, minerals, and fiber. A smoothie will help you to be more energetic during the day, thanks to the more efficient processing of its energy sources.

Also, one of the most important features is reducing toxic exposure and sugar cravings. While you consume nutritious and filling smoothies, you don't have space for other food, especially junk-food. It means that you can easily avoid processed food, doing it unconsciously because of a lack of desire and hunger. You will be surprised that you don't like McDonald's anymore.

We must consider toxic exposure as a problem as it causes food intolerances and allergies. Our body will be protected from such disease only if we enrich our daily diet with essential nutrients and reduce our intake of unhealthy sugars, fats, and preservatives. Take your diet seriously.

## REFRESH YOURSELF

With a green juice and smoothie, you will not only improve your body and immune system but also refresh your beauty. All the smoothie nutrients will make your hair glow and shine again, and your skin will look healthy and fresh. It will help you to stay hydrated longer and reduce sagging.

Remember, what you eat has a direct effect on your skin and hair. If you often eat junk food, you will notice that your skin and hair become dull-looking, unhealthy, and dehydrated.

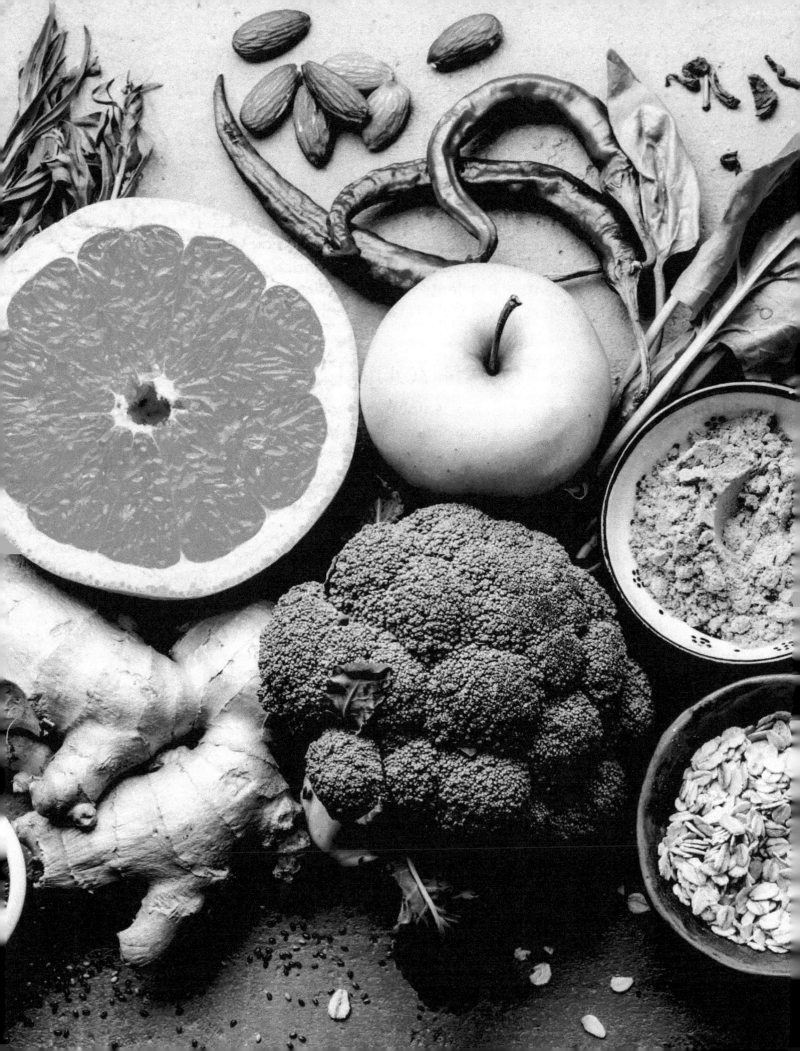

# Chapter 10

# Recipes:
# Breakfast

# 01 Sirtfood Green Onion and Mushroom Omelet

**Cooking:** 5'
**Preparation:** 10'
**Serves:** 2

## Ingredients

- 6 oz. crimini mushrooms
- 2 tbsps. Plus 2 tsps. Butter
- 5 tbsps. Chopped green onions
- 1/4 cup dry vermouth
- 6 large eggs
- 1 tbsp. water
- 1/4 tsp. salt
- 1/4 tsp. ground black pepper

## Directions

1. In processor, finely chop mushrooms. Melt 2 tbsp. butter on medium high heat in medium skillet. Add 3 tbsp. onions and mushrooms; sauté for 3 minutes.
2. Add vermouth; boil for 1 1/2 minutes till evaporated. Season with pepper and salt.
3. Whisk pepper, salt, 1 tbsp. water and eggs to blend in medium bowl. Melt 1 tsp. butter on medium heat in small nonstick skillet.
4. Add 1/2 egg mixture; mix with back of a fork till edges start to set. Cook, lifting edges using a spatula so uncooked egg flows underneath, for 2 minutes till omelet is set.
5. Put 1/2 mushroom mixture down the middle of omelet then folds both omelet sides over filling; put onto plate.
6. Repeat using leftover mushroom mixture, egg mixture and butter. Sprinkle leftover onions on omelets.

## Nutritional Facts

Calories per serving: 399; Carbohydrates: 15g; Protein: 1g; Fat: 0g; Sugar: 0.6g; Sodium: 506mg; Fiber: 1g

# 02 Sirtfood Nutmeg-Coated Creamy French Toast

COOKING: 15'
PREPARATION: 10'
SERVES: 4

## Ingredients

- One 1-lb. loaf unsliced bread, preferably challah, brioche, or another rich egg bread, or a firm, fine-textured white bread
- 5 eggs plus 3 egg yolks
- 1/4 tsp. salt
- 1 cup half-and-half or milk
- 1/2 cup plain yogurt, preferably Greek
- 3 tbsps. Granulated sugar
- 2 tsps. Ground nutmeg, plus 1/8 tsp.
- Butter or canola oil for frying
- 2 tbsps. Powdered sugar
- Maple syrup or fruit preserves for serving

## Directions

1. Cut bread to slightly less than 1-in. thick slices.
2. Put bread into a 13x9-in. pan in 1 layer; if needed, use an extra 8-in. square pan.
3. Whisk salt, egg yolks and eggs till they're fully smooth, frothy and light for 1-2 minutes in a medium bowl. You shouldn't have stringiness or egg bits left; there will be cooked egg pieces on the toast if so. Whisk in 2 tsp. nutmeg, granulated sugar, yogurt and half and half till well blended. Put egg mixture on bread. Use plastic wrap to cover; refrigerate overnight, flipping bread 1-2 times carefully if you can.
4. Heat a nonstick skillet on medium heat or preheat the electric nonstick griddle to around 350°F when ready to cook. Brush some butter on the skillet or griddle lightly; in batches, cook bread, turning once, till golden brown outside yet soft in the middle for 6-8 minutes. As needed, adjust the heat.
5. As the bread fries, mix 1/8 tsp. nutmeg and powdered sugar; put it into the fine-mesh strainer. Sprinkle the powdered sugar mixture on the hot French toast. Top with preserves or maple syrup; serve.
6. So each slice has a creamy center, the bread is sliced thickly; however, they shouldn't be too thick otherwise the center will not cook but the outside will.

## Nutritional Facts

Calories per serving: 895; Carbohydrates: 15g; Protein: 1g; Fat: 0g; Sugar: 0.6g; Sodium: 36mg; Fiber: 1g

# 03 Dried Cherry and Golden Raisin Turnovers

**Cooking:** 30'
**Preparation:** 10'
**Serves:** 4

## Ingredients

- 1 frozen puff pastry sheet (from a 17 1/4-oz package), thawed
- 3 oz. cream cheese, softened
- 2 tbsps. Sugar
- 3/4 cup mixed dried sour cherries and golden raisins
- 1 large egg, lightly beaten

## Directions

1. Preheat an oven to 400°F.
2. Use a sharp knife to quarter puff pastry to make 4 squares. Mix 1 1/2 tbsp. sugar and cream cheese; divide to squares and spread to leave 3/4-in. pastry border all around. Sprinkle cream cheese with fruit. Brush pastry border with some egg. To enclose filling, fold pastry to a triangle; use a fork to crimp edges. On tops of turnovers, cut small steam vent. Brush more egg on tops; sprinkle leftover 1 tbsp. sugar.
3. Put onto lightly buttered baking sheet; bake in lower oven third for 25 minutes till golden brown and puffed.

## Nutritional Facts

Calories per serving: 311; Carbohydrates: 49.6g; Protein: 2g; Fat: 0.4g; Sugar: 0g; Sodium: 61mg; Fiber: 1g

# 04 Sirtfood Muffins

**Cooking:** 2H15'
**Preparation:** 25'
**Serves:** 18

## Ingredients

- 1 cup milk
- 2 tbsps. White sugar
- 1 (.25 oz.) package active dry yeast
- 1 cup warm water (110 degrees F/45 degrees C)
- 1/4 cup melted shortening
- 6 cups all-purpose flour
- 1 tsp. salt

## Directions

1. In a small saucepan, warm milk until it is bubbling. Take away from the heat. Add sugar while stirring until it is dissolved. Allow cooling to lukewarm. Dissolve the yeast in warm water in a small bowl and leave to sit for about 10 minutes until creamy.
2. Combine 3 cups flour, shortening, yeast mixture, and milk in a large bowl. Then beat until the mix is smooth. Pour in salt and remaining flour or enough of it to form a soft dough. Knead and transfer into a greased bowl. Cover the dough and leave it to rise.
3. Press down and then roll out into about half inch thick. Use empty tuna can, drinking glass or a biscuit cutter to cut the rounds. Drizzle cornmeal onto waxed paper and leave the rounds to rise on this. Dust cornmeal onto the tops of muffins. Cover them and allow rising for 1/2 hour.
4. Heat griddle that is greased and then cook the muffins for about 10 minutes per side in the griddle over medium heat. Keep the baked muffins in a warm oven until all are cooked. Cool, transfer into plastic bags and store.

## Chef Tip

To use, cut and then toast. Good together with jam, cream cheese or orange butter.

## Nutritional Facts

Calories per serving: 163; Carbohydrates: 45.6 g; Protein: 3 g; Fat: 0.6g; Sugar: 1g; Sodium: 87mg; Fiber: .7 g

# 05 Baked Eggs With Cantal Cheese

**Cooking:** 15'
**Preparation:** 25'
**Serves:** 6

## Ingredients

- Butter for greasing ramekins
- 6 large eggs
- 1/4 tsp. salt
- 1/4 tsp. black pepper
- 1/8 tsp. freshly grated nutmeg
- 1/8 tsp. cream of tartar
- 3 oz. coarsely grated Cantal cheese (1 cup)
- 6 tbsps. Crème fraîche
- 1 tbsp. chopped fresh chives
- 6 (8-oz) ramekins or a 13- by 9- by 2-inch baking dish

## Directions

1. Put oven rack into center position; preheat an oven to 350°F and butter baking dish/ramekins.
2. Separate eggs, carefully sliding unbroken, whole yolks into small bowl with cold water and putting whites into a big bowl.
3. Use an electric mixer on medium-high speed to beat whites with cream of tartar, nutmeg, pepper and salt till they hold stiff peaks; gently yet thoroughly fold in 1/2 cup of cheese. Divide it to ramekins or put it into a baking dish, slightly smoothing top (whites stand above the ramekin's rims). Make 6 evenly spaced indentations for baking dish or indentation in middle of whites in every ramekin. One by one, use your fingers to remove yolks from water carefully; in each indentation, put 1 yolk.
4. Mix crème Fraiche; put 1 tbsp. over each yolk. Sprinkle leftover cheese on eggs. If using, put ramekins onto big shallow baking pan.
5. Bake for 10-14 minutes till whites are pale golden and puffed (yolks will slightly jiggly). Sprinkle chives; immediately serve.

## Chef Tip

Be aware the yolks aren't fully cooked in this recipe; it can be an issue if salmonella is common in your area. Bake eggs till yolks set if desired.

## Nutritional Facts

Calories per serving: 164; Carbohydrates: 33g; Protein: 1.4g; Fat: 2g; Sugar: 0.3g; Sodium: 43mg; Fiber: 1g

# Chapter 11

# Recipes:
# Salads

# 06 Sirtfood Green Salad

**Cooking:** 30'
**Preparation:** 15'
**Serves:** 8

## Ingredients

- 1/2 cup chopped onion
- 1/2 cup chopped green bell pepper
- 2 (10 oz.) packages mixed salad greens
- 4 thinly sliced chicken deli meat, chopped
- 1 tomato, chopped
- 1/4 tsp. onion powder
- 3 dashes garlic powder
- 1 pinch ground black pepper
- 2 pinches salt
- 3 tbsps. Balsamic vinaigrette salad dressing

## Directions

1. Sauté or microwave bell pepper and onion till softened then put aside, let cool.
2. Combine tomato, deli meat, salad greens, pepper and onion in a large salad bowl. Sprinkle salt, black pepper, garlic powder and onion powder over. Toss till mixed.
3. Add enough vinegar or salad dressing to coat. Toss again to serve.

## Nutritional Facts

Calories per serving: 118; Carbohydrates: 65g; Protein: 1.8g; Fat: 2g; Sugar: 0.3g; Sodium: 72mg; Fiber: 0g

# 07 Sirtfood Layered Taco Salad

**Cooking:** 45'
**Preparation:** 45'
**Serves:** 6

## Ingredients

- 1/4 cup fresh lime juice
- 1/2 cup chopped fresh cilantro
- 1 tsp. sugar
- 1 tbsp. chili powder
- 1/4 tsp. ground cumin
- 1/2 tsp. salt
- 1/4 tsp. black pepper
- 1/2 cup olive oil
- 1 medium onion, chopped
- 3 garlic cloves, finely chopped
- 1 to 2 fresh Serrano chiles (including seeds), finely chopped
- 1 tbsp. chili powder
- 2 tsps. Ground cumin
- 2 tbsps. Olive oil
- 1 1/2 lb. ground chuck
- 1 (8-oz) can tomato sauce
- 1/2 tsp. salt
- 1/4 tsp. black pepper
- 1 (1/2-lb) firm-ripe California avocado
- 1 head iceberg lettuce, thinly sliced (8 cups)
- 1 large tomato (1/2 lb.), chopped
- 1/4 lb. coarsely grated extra-sharp Cheddar (1 1/2 cups)
- 1 (15- to 19-oz) can black beans, drained and rinsed
- 1 (6-oz) can sliced pitted California black olives, drained
- Accompaniment: tortilla chips

## Directions

1. <u>For the dressing:</u> Mix chili powder, salt, lime juice, pepper, cumin, cilantro, and sugar. Add oil gradually in a stream, mix until the mixture emulsified.
2. For the beef: Heat oil in a 12-inch heavy skillet over medium heat. Cook cumin, garlic, chili powder, onion, and chilies to taste for 6 minutes, stirring it for some time until the onion is tender. Stir in beef and cook for 5 minutes, stirring and breaking up the lumps until the meat is no longer pink. Remove any excess fat from skillet.
3. Pour tomato sauce, pepper, and salt into the browned beef and cook for 3 minutes, stirring it frequently until slightly thickened. Remove the mixture from heat.

4. <u>For the salad:</u> Peel and pit the avocado and cut into halves. Slice it into 1/2-inch pieces.
5. In a shallow 4-qt dish, arrange the lettuce over the bottom. Pour the beef mixture evenly on top of the lettuce.
6. Make another layer on top by arranging avocado, beans, olives, cheese, and tomatoes. Spread the dressing all over the salad.

**NUTRITIONAL FACTS** Calories per serving: 330; Carbohydrates: 54g; Protein: 1.2g; Fat: 1g; Sugar: 0.4g; Sodium: 86mg; Fiber: 0g

# 08 Cucumber Fennel Salad

**Cooking:** 20'
**Preparation:** 20'
**Serves:** 8

## Ingredients

- 3 large cucumbers, sliced
- 1 medium sweet onion, thinly sliced
- 1 small fennel bulb, thinly sliced
- 3 tbsps. Lemon juice
- 3 tbsps. Olive oil
- 3/4 tsp. dill weeds
- 1/2 tsp. salt
- 1/4 tsp. pepper
- 1/4 tsp. grated lemon peel

## Directions

1. Mix fennel, onion, and cucumber together in a big bowl. In a tightly fitting lidded jar, mix the rest of the ingredients together; shake well.
2. Put on the cucumber mixture and mix to combine. Put in the fridge until cold.

## Nutritional Facts

Calories per serving: 335; Carbohydrates: 21g; Protein: 3g; Fat: 1g; Sugar: 0.6g; Sodium: 202mg; Fiber: 1g

# 09 Sirtfood Apple Coleslaw

**Cooking:** 8H15'
**Preparation:** 15'
**Serves:** 6

## Ingredients

- 4 cups shredded cabbage
- 1 cup shredded carrot
- 1 Granny Smith apple – peeled, cored and coarsely shredded
- 2 tbsps. Honey
- 1 tbsp. brown sugar
- 2 tsps. White vinegar
- 1 tbsp. pineapple juice (optional)
- 2 tbsps. Mayonnaise
- 1 dash salt
- 1 tsp. ground black pepper

## Directions

1. Toss sliced apple, carrot, and shredded cabbage together in a bowl. Mix mayonnaise, honey, pineapple juice, brown sugar, and vinegar together in another bowl until the sugar and honey dissolves.
2. Toss the cabbage mix and dressing together until well coated. Sprinkle pepper and salt; mix and cover.
3. Refrigerate until ready to use.

## Nutritional Facts

Calories per serving: 240; Carbohydrates: 33.7g; Protein: 5g; Fat: 2g; Sugar: 0.5g; Sodium: 87mg; Fiber: 1g

# 10 Carrot Bean Salad

**Cooking:** 20'
**Preparation:** 20'
**Serves:** 6

## Ingredients

- 2 cups thinly sliced carrots
- 1 cans (15 oz.) garbanzo beans or chickpeas, rinsed and drained
- 1 cup thinly sliced celery
- 2 tbsps. Lemon juice
- 2 tsps. Olive oil
- 1/2 tsp. lemon-pepper seasoning
- 1/4 tsp. salt
- 1/2 cup minced fresh cilantro

## Directions

1. In a steamer basket, add carrots; set in a saucepan over 1 inch of water.
2. Boil; put a cover on and steam until crisp-tender, 5-6 minutes. Immediately put the carrots in ice water in a bowl.
3. Mix celery and garbanzo beans together in a separate bowl. Drain the carrots and put in the bean mixture.
4. Combine salt, lemon-pepper, oil, and lemon juice in a small bowl. Add onto the carrot mixture and toss until coated. Put a cover on and chill for a minimum of 4 hours.
5. Mix in cilantro right before eating.

## Nutritional Facts

Calories per serving: 154; Carbohydrates: 29.8g; Protein: 2g; Fat: 1g; Sugar: 0.5g; Sodium: 98mg; Fiber: 1g

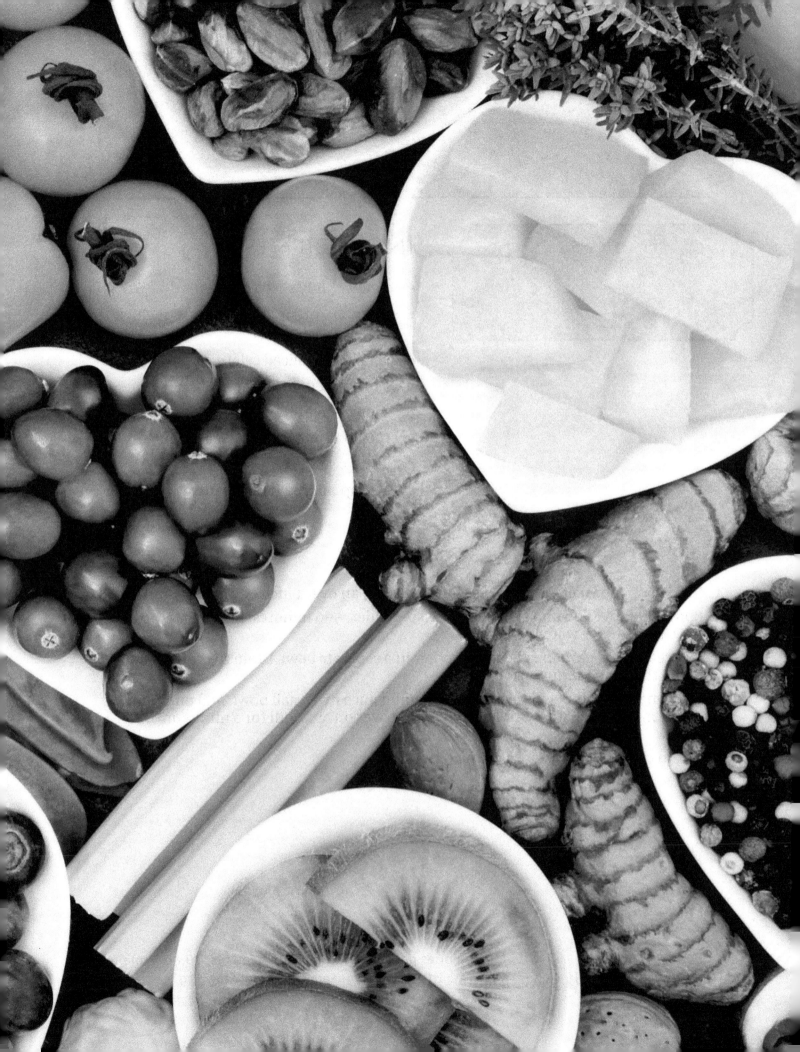

# Chapter 12

# Recipes:
# Meat

# 11 Sirtfood Pork Roast

**COOKING:** 5-7H
**PREPARATION:** 5'
**SERVES:** 4-6

## INGREDIENTS

- 2 apples, cored, peeled, and sliced
- 2 garlic cloves, peeled
- 2 tablespoons apple cider
- 1½ cups water
- Salt and pepper to taste
- ½ teaspoon ground ginger
- ¼ cup all-purpose flour
- 1 (3-pound) pork loin roast
- 2 teaspoons oil
- 1 stalk celery, roughly chopped
- 4 large carrots, roughly chopped
- 1 onion, sliced (divided)

## DIRECTIONS

1. Combine ¼ of the onion, ½ of the apple slices, and the garlic in a food processor. Process to a very smooth consistency.
2. Pour the mixture into the slow cooker, and then add the apple cider and water.
3. Combine the salt, pepper, ginger and flour in a large shallow bowl. Roll the pork loin in the flour mixture, pressing gently to coat all sides.
4. Heat the oil over medium-high heat in a large skillet. Sear the coated roast on all sides, and then transfer it to the slow cooker. Add the remaining vegetables, onion and apple slices.
5. Cover and cook on low for about 6–7 hours or until the roast is completely cooked through.
6. Serve topped with the juices from the slow cooker.

## NUTRITIONAL FACTS

Calories: 567; Fat: 34 g; Carbs: 52 g; Protein: 4 g
Sodium: 933 g

# 12 Sirtfood Fried Chicken

COOKING: 30'
PREPARATION: 15'
SERVES: 4

## Ingredients

- Chicken
- ½ cup all-purpose flour
- 1 teaspoon poultry seasoning
- ½ teaspoon salt
- ½ teaspoon pepper
- 1 egg, slightly beaten
- 1 tablespoon water
- 4 boneless skinless chicken breasts, pounded to ½-inch thickness
- 1 cup vegetable oil
- Gravy
- 2 tablespoons all-purpose flour
- ¼ teaspoon salt
- ¼ teaspoon pepper
- 1¼ cups milk

## Directions

1. Preheat the oven to 200°F.
2. In a shallow dish, combine the flour, poultry seasoning, salt and pepper.
3. In another shallow dish, mix together the beaten egg and water.
4. First dip both sides of the chicken breasts in the flour mixture, then dip them in the egg mixture, and then back into the flour mixture.
5. Heat the vegetable oil over medium-high heat in a large deep skillet. A cast iron is good choice if you have one. Add the chicken and cook for about 15 minutes or until fully cooked, turning over about halfway through.
6. Transfer the chicken to a cookie sheet and place in the oven to maintain temperature.
7. Remove all but 2 tablespoons of oil from the skillet you cooked the chicken in.
8. Prepare the gravy by whisking the dry gravy ingredients together in a bowl. Then whisk them into the oil in the skillet, stirring thoroughly to remove lumps. When the flour begins to brown, slowly whisk in the milk. Continue cooking and whisking for about 2 minutes or until the mixture thickens.
9. Top chicken with some of the gravy.

## Nutritional Facts

Calories: 634; Fat: 24 g ; Carbs: 54 g; Protein: 61 g; Sodium: 1286 mg

# 13 Sirtfood Steak Diane

**COOKING:** 15'
**PREPARATION:** 10'
**SERVES:** 2

## Ingredients

- 2–3 tablespoons butter
- 12 ounces beef tenderloin, cut into 3-ounce medallions
- Salt to taste
- 2 teaspoons cracked whole black peppercorns
- ½ cup fresh mushrooms, sliced
- 3 tablespoons pearl onions, chopped
- ¼ cup brandy or white wine
- 1 teaspoon Worcestershire sauce
- 1 tablespoon Dijon mustard
- ¾ cup beef stock
- ¼ cup cream

## Directions

1. Preheat the oven to 350°F.
2. In a large skillet, melt 2 tablespoons of the butter over medium-high heat.
3. Sprinkle both sides of the beef medallions with salt and fresh pepper. Sear them for about 2 minutes on each side, and then remove them from the skillet to an ovenproof dish and transfer it to the oven to keep warm.
4. While those are in the oven, add a bit more butter to the skillet. Add the mushrooms and pearl onions and cook until they start to turn soft. Add the white wine and Worcestershire, and then stir in the mustard. Cook for about 2 minutes.
5. Stir in the beef stock and bring it to a boil. When it boils, remove it from the heat and stir in the cream.
6. Remove the beef from the oven and plate it with sauce

## Nutritional Facts

Calories: 421; Fat: 31 g; Carbs: 24 g; Protein: 43 g; Sodium: 1354 mg

# 14 Turkey Sandwich

COOKING: 8'
PREPARATION: 10'
SERVES: 1

## Ingredients

- 2 slices Italian bread
- 1 Tbsp. CLASSICO Traditional Basil Pesto Sauce and Spread
- 6 slices OSCAR MAYER Deli Fresh Honey Smoked Turkey Breast
- 1 KRAFT Provolone Cheese Slice
- 2 small pepperoncini peppers, stemmed, sliced
- 1-1/2 tsp. chopped black olives

## Directions

1. Spread bread slices with pesto; fill with remaining ingredients.2
2. Heat small skillet sprayed with cooking spray on medium heat.3
3. Add sandwich; cook 4 min. on each side or until golden brown on both sides.

## Nutritional Facts

Calories: 350; Fat: 15g; Carbs: 33g; Fibers: 2g; Sugar: 2g; Protein: 22g;

# 15 Taco Bell Spicy Tostada

**Cooking:** 15'
**Preparation:** 15'
**Serves:** 4

## Ingredients

- 1/2 pound lean ground beef (90% lean)
- 1 can (10 ounces) diced tomatoes and green chilies, undrained
- 1 can (15 ounces) black beans, rinsed and drained
- 1 can (16 ounces) refried beans, warmed
- 8 tostada shells
- Optional toppings: shredded reduced-fat Mexican cheese blend, shredded lettuce, salsa and sour cream

## Directions

1. In a large skillet, cook and crumble beef over medium-high heat until no longer pink, 4-6 minutes. Stir in tomatoes; bring to a boil. Reduce heat; simmer, uncovered, until liquid is almost evaporated, 6-8 minutes. Stir in black beans; heat through.
2. To serve, spread refried beans over tostada shells. Top with beef mixture; add toppings as desired.

## Nutritional Facts

Calories: 559; Fats: 14g; Carbs: 46g; Sugars: 2g; Fiber: 10g; Protein: 23g

# Chapter 13

# Recipes:
# Fish

# 16 Sirtfood Crusty Fish Fillets

**COOKING:** 25'
**PREPARATION:** 15'
**SERVES:** 4

## Ingredients

- ¼ cup toasted wheat germ
- 2 tbsps. Finely chopped pecans
- 1 tbsp. finely chopped fresh parsley
- 1 clove garlic, minced
- ¼ tsp. salt
- ⅛ Tsp. cayenne pepper
- 4 4-oz. fish fillets, such as catfish or Pacific flounder

## Directions

1. Start preheating the oven to 425°F. Grease a baking sheet with cooking spray.
2. Mix cayenne, salt, garlic, parsley, pecans, and wheat germ in a pie pan. Dredge fillets in the wheat germ mixture. Arrange on the greased baking sheet and bake for 12 to 15 minutes until the center is opaque.
3. Serve with lemon wedges.

## Nutritional Facts

Calories per serving: 133; Carbohydrates: 34g; Protein: 3g; Fat: 1g; Sugar: 2g; Sodium: 72mg; Fiber: 0g

# 17 Garlic Anchovy Linguine

Cooking: 40'
Preparation: 20'
Serves: 6

## Ingredients

- 6 tbsps. Extra-virgin olive oil
- 6 cloves garlic, chopped
- 3/4 cup finely chopped broccoli florets
- 1/2 cup sliced mushrooms
- 6 oz. anchovy fillets, chopped
- 1 cup water
- 1/4 cup chopped green onions
- 1/2 cup diced tomatoes
- 2 tbsps. Finely chopped fresh parsley
- 1 tsp. extra-virgin olive oil
- 1 (16 oz.) package linguine pasta
- 1 1/2 tbsps. Crushed red pepper flakes
- 1 pinch black pepper (optional)

## Directions

1. Heat 6 tbsp. of olive oil in a big skillet on medium heat. Mix in mushrooms, broccoli and garlic; cook till browned lightly. Add water and anchovies; cover.
2. Simmer for 4-5 minutes.
3. Mix in parsley, tomatoes and green onions; cover.
4. Simmer for 3-4 minutes till veggies are soft.
5. Boil 1 tsp. of olive oil and a big pot of water as veggies cook. Add linguine; cook for 7-8 minutes till al dente; drain. Toss with crushed red pepper flakes and anchovy mixture; season with black pepper if preferred. Immediately serve.
6. Drizzle honey over sandwiches and put a fried egg on top of each.

## Nutritional Facts

Calories per serving: 195; Carbohydrates: 37g; Protein: 1.4g; Fat: 34g; Sugar: 3g; Sodium: 58mg; Fiber: 0g

# 18 Tuna & Bok Choy Packets

**Cooking:** 30'
**Preparation:** 15'
**Serves:** 4

## Ingredients

- ¼ cup horseradish mustard
- ¼ cup finely chopped parsley, divided
- 2 tbsps. Water
- ¼ tsp. freshly ground pepper
- 2 baby bok choy, trimmed and quartered lengthwise
- 1 tbsp. extra-virgin olive oil
- 1-1¼ lbs. tuna, wild salmon, mahi-mahi or cod, skinned if desired, cut into 4 portions

## Directions

1. Preheat the oven to 475°F. In a small bowl, mix the pepper, water, 3 tbsps. Of parsley and mustard together.
2. In a big bowl, mix 2 tbsps. Of mustard sauce, oil and boy choy together by tossing.
3. Get the foil ready by cutting four sheets of them up, around 20 inches each. In the middle of every piece, set 2 bok choy quarters down. Over the top of the vegetables, put a tbsp. of the leftover sauce after putting a portion of fish atop. Seal the packets up by bringing the foils' short ends together then folding them over and pinching the side seams. Put them on top of a very big baking sheet. Depending on how thick the fish is, bake for around 15 minutes or more until the center turns opaque. Be very careful of the steam that will escape when you unseal the packet to see if the fish is done. Scatter the leftover tbsp. of parsley atop before serving.

## Nutritional Facts

Calories per serving: 146; Carbohydrates: 6g; Protein: 4.5g; Fat: 4g; Sugar: 3g; Sodium: 48mg; Fiber: 0g

# 19 Sirtfood Caramel Coated Catfish

**Cooking:** 45'
**Preparation:** 15'
**Serves:** 4

## Ingredients

- 1/3 cup water
- 2 tbsps. Fish sauce
- 2 shallots, chopped
- 4 cloves garlic, minced
- 1 1/2 tsps. Ground black pepper
- 1/4 tsp. red pepper flakes
- 1/3 cup water
- 1/3 cup white sugar
- 2 lbs. catfish fillets
- 1/2 tsp. white sugar
- 1 tbsp. fresh lime juice
- 1 green onion, thinly sliced
- 1/2 cup chopped cilantro

## Directions

1. Combine fish sauce and 1/3 cup of water in a small bowl; mix and put aside.
2. Combine together shallots, red pepper flakes, black pepper and garlic in another bowl and put aside.
3. Heat 1/3 cup of sugar and 1/3 cup of water in a big skillet placed over medium heat, stirring from time to time until sugar becomes deep golden brown. Stir in the fish sauce mixture gently and let the mixture boil. Mix and cook the shallot mixture.
4. Once the shallots have softened, add the catfish to the mixture.
5. Cook the catfish with cover for about 5 minutes each side until the fish can be easily flake using a fork. Transfer the catfish to a large plate, place a cover, and put aside. Adjust the heat to high and mix in a half tsp. of sugar.
6. Stir in any sauce that left on the plate and the lime juice.
7. Let it boil and simmer until the sauce has cooked down.
8. Drizzle the sauce on top of the catfish and sprinkle with cilantro and green onions.

## Nutritional Facts

Calories per serving: 254; Carbohydrates: 4g; Protein: 1g; Fat: 0.5g; Sugar: 3g; Sodium: 96mg; Fiber: 1g

# 20 New Orleans Stuffed Artichokes

**Cooking:** 30'
**Preparation:** 3H45'
**Serves:** 10

## Ingredients

- 10 whole artichokes
- 1 cup Italian seasoned bread crumbs
- 4 oz. provolone cheese, shredded
- 10 pimento-stuffed green olives, chopped
- 1/2 bunch fresh parsley, chopped
- 5 cloves garlic, minced
- 1 bunch green onions, finely chopped
- 2 small stalks celery, finely chopped
- 1/2 green bell pepper, finely chopped
- 1 tsp. lemon juice
- 1 tsp. hot pepper sauce (e.g. Tabasco™)
- 4 (2 oz.) cans anchovy fillets, chopped
- 1 tsp. Worcestershire sauce
- 1 tbsp. olive oil, or as needed
- Salt to taste

## Directions

1. To prepare artichokes, cut off the bottoms of stems and trim the tips of leaves. To trim leaves, scissors is the best choice. Tear off small leaves around base and throw them away.
2. In a big pot, add artichokes and enough amount of water to cover. On top of them, put a dinner plate to prevent the artichokes from floating out of water. Place a lid on pot to cover and bring to a boil. Boil until there are some leaves floating in the water, about 10-15 minutes, then drain and cool artichokes.
3. Combine bell pepper, celery, green onions, garlic, parsley, olives, cheese and bread crumbs together in a medium bowl. Stir salt, olive oil, Worcestershire sauce, anchovies, hot pepper sauce and lemon juice together in a small bowl, then stir into the bread crumb mixture.
4. Tear off a big square of aluminum foil for each artichoke. Put one artichoke in the center of each square and tuck approximately 1/2 tsp. of the cheese mixture under each leaf. Gather up foil around artichoke and leave top opening.
5. In bottom of a big pot, set a wire rack or steamer insert, then fill with 3 in. of fresh water or so that artichokes remain above water level. Place artichokes upright in the pot and bring to a boil. Place on a cover and allow artichokes to steam about 3 hours. Take out of the pot and let them cool to room temperature prior to serving.

## Nutritional Facts

Calories per serving: 562; Carbohydrates: 52g; Protein: 3g; Fat: 3.4g; Sugar: 1g; Sodium: 77mg; Fiber: 0g

# Chapter 14

# Recipes:
# Soups

# 21 Sirtfood Beef Tortellini Soup

**Cooking:** 1H20'
**Preparation:** 15'
**Serves:** 12

## Ingredients

- 1 lb. ground beef
- 7 cups beef broth
- 2 cans (14-1/2 oz. each) stewed tomatoes
- 3/4 cup ketchup
- 3/4 cup thinly sliced carrots
- 3/4 cup thinly sliced celery
- 3/4 cup finely chopped onion
- 1 tbsp. dried basil
- 1-1/2 tsps. Seasoned salt
- 1 tsp. sugar
- 1/4 tsp. pepper
- 4 bay leaves
- 1-1/2 cups frozen cheese tortellini
- Grated Parmesan cheese, optional

## Directions

1. Brown beef in a soup kettle or Dutch oven; let drain. Add the following 11 ingredients; boil up. Then lower heat; cover and stew for 30 minutes.
2. Put in tortellini; cook until tender, about 20-30 minutes more. Discard the bay leaves. If desired, garnish each serving with Parmesan cheese.

## Nutritional Facts

Calories per serving: 267; Carbohydrates: 34g; Protein: 0.5g; Fat: 0.4g; Sugar: 2g; Sodium: 37mg; Fiber: 0g

# 22 Sirtfood Meat and Potato Soup

**Cooking:** 30'
**Preparation:** 15'
**Serves:** 6

## Ingredients

- 4 cups water
- 3 cups cubed cooked beef chuck roast
- 4 medium red potatoes, cubed
- 4 oz. sliced fresh mushrooms
- 1/2 cup chopped onion
- 1/4 cup ketchup
- 2 tsps. Beef bouillon granules
- 2 tsps. Cider vinegar
- 1 tsp. brown sugar
- 1 tsp. Worcestershire sauce
- 1/8 tsp. ground mustard
- 1 cup coarsely chopped fresh spinach

## Directions

1. Slice leeks into thin slices. Sauté onion and leeks in butter in a skillet until softened but not browned. Pour into a Dutch oven or soup kettle.
2. Add parsley, broth, add potatoes; simmer, covered until vegetables are tender. Drain; put broth aside. Transfer vegetables to a food processor or blender and process into puree. Pour the puree and broth back to the pan. Add a small amount of pureed mixture into egg yolk; pour back into the pan. Put in nutmeg, pepper, and salt. Cook the mixture over medium heat, stirring from time to time, until it reaches 160° on a thermometer.
3. Mix in cream. Cook until thoroughly heated (without boiling). Top with bacon to garnish.

## Nutritional Facts

Calories per serving: 255; Carbohydrates: 3g; Protein: 1g; Fat: 6g; Sugar: 0.6g; Sodium: 283mg; Fiber: 1g

# 23 Leek Soup

**COOKING:** 30'
**PREPARATION:** 30'
**SERVES:** 12

## Ingredients

- 6 wild leeks
- 1 medium onion, thinly sliced
- 1/4 cup butter, cubed
- 6 medium potatoes, peeled and sliced
- 6 cups chicken broth
- 1/2 cup minced fresh parsley
- 1 egg yolk, beaten
- 1-1/2 tsps. Salt
- 1/4 tsp. pepper
- Pinch ground nutmeg
- 2 cups half-and-half cream
- 4 bacon strips, cooked and crumbled

## Directions

1. Slice leeks into thin slices. Sauté onion and leeks in butter in a skillet until softened but not browned. Pour into a Dutch oven or soup kettle.
2. Add parsley, broth, add potatoes; simmer, covered until vegetables are tender. Drain; put broth aside. Transfer vegetables to a food processor or blender and process into puree. Pour the puree and broth back to the pan. Add a small amount of pureed mixture into egg yolk; pour back into the pan. Put in nutmeg, pepper, and salt. Cook the mixture over medium heat, stirring from time to time, until it reaches 160° on a thermometer.
3. Mix in cream. Cook until thoroughly heated (without boiling). Top with bacon to garnish.

## Nutritional Facts

Calories per serving: 204; Carbohydrates: 43g; Protein: 1.5g; Fat: 2g; Sugar: 0.3g; Sodium: 86mg; Fiber: 3g

# 24 Chicken 'n' Dumpling Soup

Cooking: 35'
Preparation: 2H20'
Serves: 20

## Ingredients

- 1 broiler/fryer chicken (3 to 3-1/2 lbs.)
- 3 quarts water
- 1/4 cup chicken bouillon granules
- 1 bay leaf
- 1 tsp. whole peppercorns
- 1/8 tsp. ground allspice
- 6 cups uncooked wide noodles
- 4 cups sliced carrots
- 1 package (10 oz.) frozen mixed vegetables
- 3/4 cup sliced celery
- 1/2 cup chopped onion
- 1/4 cup uncooked long grain rice
- 2 tbsps. Minced fresh parsley
- DUMPLINGS:
- 1-1/3 cups all-purpose flour
- 2 tsps. Baking powder
- 1 tsp. dried thyme
- 1/2 tsp. salt
- 2/3 cup milk
- 2 tbsps. Canola oil

## Directions

1. Mix the initial 6 ingredients together in a stockpot; heat to a boil. Decrease the heat and let simmer for 1-1/2 hours with cover. Take out chicken, let cool down. Strain broth; get rid of peppercorns and bay leaf.
2. Take bones out of chicken, get rid of bones. Chop meat into bite-size chunks. Bring broth back to the pan and skim fat. Put in parsley, rice, vegetables, noodles, and chicken; heat to a simmer.
3. To make dumplings, in a bowl, mix together salt, thyme, baking powder, and flour. Blend oil and milk then combine with dry ingredients. Drop into the simmering soup, by teaspoonful. Decrease the heat; simmer 15 minutes with cover (do not open cover when simmering).

## Nutritional Facts

Calories per serving: 63; Carbohydrates: 12g; Protein: 1g; Fat: 1g; Sugar: 0.5g; Sodium: 36mg; Fiber: 0g

# 25 Sirtfood Sausage Cabbage Soup

**Cooking:** 40'
**Preparation:** 20'
**Serves:** 6

## Ingredients

- 1 medium onion, chopped
- 1 tbsp. canola oil
- 1 tbsp. butter
- 2 medium carrots, thinly sliced and halved
- 1 celery rib, thinly sliced
- 1 tsp. caraway seeds
- 2 cups water
- 2 cups chopped cabbage
- 1/2 lb. fully cooked Johnsonville® Fully Cooked Polish Kielbasa Sausage Rope, halved and cut into 1/4-inch slices
- 1 can (14-1/2 oz.) diced tomatoes, undrained
- 1 tbsp. brown sugar
- 1 can (15 oz.) white kidney beans, rinsed and drained
- 1 tbsp. white vinegar
- 1 tsp. salt
- 1/4 tsp. pepper
- Minced fresh parsley

## Directions

1. Sauté onion in butter and oil in a 3-qt. saucepan until it becomes tender. Mix in carrots and celery and cook for 3 minutes. Put in caraway and cook, stirring continuously, for 1 more minute. Mix in the brown sugar, tomatoes, sausage, cabbage, and water and let it boil. Adjust heat. Simmer while covered for 15-20 minutes until veggies become tender.
2. Put in the pepper, salt, vinegar and beans. Take out the cover and simmer for 5-10 minutes until it is heated through. Drizzle with parsley.

## Nutritional Facts

Calories per serving: 486; Carbohydrates: 34g; Protein: 2g; Fat: 0.7g; Sugar: 1g; Sodium: 65mg; Fiber: 0g

# Chapter 15

# Recipes:
# Sacks

# 26 Sirtfood Cheddar Crackers

**Cooking:** 55'
**Preparation:** 15'
**Serves:** 48

## Ingredients

- 2 cups all-purpose flour
- 1 tsp. salt
- 1/4 tsp. ground white pepper
- 1/4 tsp. dry mustard
- 3/4 cup butter, chilled
- 1/2 cup shredded Cheddar cheese
- 6 tbsps. Cold water, or as needed

## Directions

1. Mix flour, mustard, salt, and white pepper in a medium bowl. Use a fork to cut in the butter until the mixture looks like coarse crumbs. Mix in Cheddar cheese. Pour in water, 1 tbsp. at a time, until the dough can hold together. Form the mixture into a ball. Wrap it and store it inside the fridge for at least 30 minutes.
2. Set the oven to 350°F or 175°C for preheating. Use a parchment paper to line the baking sheets.
3. Roll out dough into the lightly floured surface and form it into a 16x12-inches rectangle with a thickness of about 1/8-inch. Cut the dough into 1x3-inches strips. Arrange the strips about 1-inch apart from each other into the prepared baking sheets.
4. In the preheated oven, bake the strips for 10-12 minutes or until crispy and golden. Let them cool completely before storing.

## Nutritional Facts

Calories per serving: 437; Carbohydrates: 60g; Protein: 2g; Fat: 0.5g; Sugar: 2.3g; Sodium: 70mg; Fiber: 0g

# 27 Honey-Peanut Popcorn

**Cooking:** 5'
**Preparation:** 5'
**Serves:** 1

## Ingredients

- 3 cups air-popped popcorn
- 1 tbsp. salted peanuts
- 1 tsp. melted butter
- 1 tsp. honey

## Directions

1. In a medium bowl, mix together the peanuts and popcorn.
2. In a small bowl, whisk the honey and butter and drizzle it on top of the popcorn.

## Nutritional Facts

Calories per serving: 258; Carbohydrates: 43g; Protein: 2g; Fat: 1.9g; Sugar: 2g; Sodium: 40mg; Fiber: 1g

# 28 Lovage Pesto

**Cooking:** 10'
**Preparation:** 10'
**Serves:** 20

## Ingredients

- 1 stalk green garlic (see Tip) or 2 large cloves garlic
- ½ cup Marcona almonds
- 3 cups loosely packed fresh lovage
- 1 cup extra-virgin olive oil, divided
- ¼ cup fresh basil
- ¼ cup grated Parmesan or pecorino cheese
- ½ tsp. lemon zest
- 2 tbsps. Lemon juice
- 1 tsp. salt
- ½ tsp. ground pepper

## Directions

1. In a food processor, pulse almonds and garlic together until coarsely chopped; scrape down the sides of the processor once.
2. Put in cheese, lovage, basil, and half cup oil; blend until coarsely chopped.
3. Put in the remaining half cup of oil, lemon zest, pepper, lemon juice, and salt. Blend until coarsely chopped, scrape down the sides of the processor 1-2 times. Set aside for half an hour. Serve.

## Nutritional Facts

Calories per serving: 503; Carbohydrates: 47g; Protein: 1g; Fat: 23g; Sugar: 3g; Sodium: 58mg; Fiber: 0g

# 29 Sirtfood Mac 'n Cheese Bites

**Cooking:** 19'
**Preparation:** 15'
**Serves:** 16

## Ingredients

- 2 tsps. Butter
- 1 cup cooked macaroni
- 2 slices American cheese, diced
- 2 tbsps. Milk
- 16 thin pretzel crackers (such as Snack Factory® Pretzel Crisps®)
- 1 (4 oz.) precooked smoked sausage, cut into sixteen 1/4-inch slices
- Ground black pepper to taste

## Directions

1. In a saucepan, melt butter over medium-low heat. Sauté American cheese and macaroni in melted butter for about 2 minutes until cheese is mainly melted. Turn heat to low; stir in milk.
2. Position the oven rack about 6 inches away from the heat source and turn the oven to low broil setting. Line parchment paper over a baking sheet.
3. Arrange pretzels crackers on the prepared baking sheet; place a slice of sausage atop each cracker. Ladle 1 tbsp. of mac and cheese mixture atop sausage. Sprinkle top with black pepper.
4. Bake for 1 to 2 minutes in the preheated broiler until the pretzels and American cheese begins to brown.

## Nutritional Facts

Calories per serving: 144; Carbohydrates: 36g; Protein: 3g; Fat: 0.5g; Sugar: 2g; Sodium: 21mg; Fiber: 0.7g

# 30 Norwegian Flat Bread

**Cooking:** 30'
**Preparation:** 30'
**Serves:** 12

## Ingredients

- 1 1/3 cups whole wheat flour
- 1 1/3 cups all-purpose flour
- 1/4 cup vegetable oil
- 1 tsp. baking soda
- 1/2 tsp. salt
- 3/4 cup buttermilk, room temperature

## Directions

1. Combine salt, baking soda, oil, all-purpose flour, and whole wheat flour in a large mixing bowl. Pour in enough butter milk to assemble a stiff dough.
2. Knead dough on a well-floured work surface for half a minute.
3. Cover the dough to avoid drying. Shape a quarter cup of dough into balls and press into flat round. Flatten dough into circles of 10-inch in diameter with a rolling pin. Arrange on an unoiled cookie sheet. Run a knife along but not through the dough to score pieces into pie shapes. Do the same with the remainder of dough.
4. Bake for 8 to 10 minutes in a 350F° (175°C) oven. Transfer to a wire cooling rack and allow cooling slightly before breaking along scored lines.

## Nutritional Facts

Calories per serving: 92; Carbohydrates: 17g; Protein: 4g; Fat: 2g; Sugar: 0.9g; Sodium: 207mg; Fiber: 0g

# Chapter 16

# Recipes:
# Spreads and Dips

# 31 Brownie Batter Bean Dip

**Cooking:** 10'
**Preparation:** 10'
**Serves:** 20

## Ingredients

- 1 (16 oz.) can BUSH'S® Black Beans, rinsed and drained
- 1/2 cup packed brown sugar
- 1/2 cup unsweetened cocoa powder
- 1/2 cup almond butter
- 1/4 cup unsweetened almond milk, or more as needed
- Fresh fruit (apples, berries, pears) or graham crackers, for dipping

## Directions

1. Process almond butter, cocoa powder, brown sugar and beans till combined well in a food processor/blender. 1 tbsp. at a time, add almond milk in the blender while running till you get a spreadable and smooth consistency.
2. Serve with fresh fruit or graham crackers for dipping.

## Nutritional Facts

Calories per serving: 548; Carbohydrates: 64g; Protein: 5g; Fat: 2g; Sugar: 1g; Sodium: 64mg; Fiber: 3g

# 32 Sirtfood Artichoke and Egg Spread

**Cooking:** 10'
**Preparation:** 10'
**Serves:** 10

## Ingredients

- 1 (14 oz.) can artichoke hearts, drained and chopped
- 1/2 cup mayonnaise
- 1/2 cup sour cream
- 3 hard-boiled eggs, chopped
- 1/2 tsp. curry powder, or to taste
- Salt and ground black pepper to taste

## Directions

1. Mix black pepper, salt, curry powder, eggs, sour cream, mayonnaise, and artichoke hearts well in a bowl.

## Nutritional Facts

Calories per serving: 271; Carbohydrates: 7g; Protein: 0.7g; Fat: 2g; Sugar: 0.5g; Sodium: 36mg; Fiber: 1g

# 33 Spinach and Artichoke Dip

**Cooking:** 25'
**Preparation:** 10'
**Serves:** 6

## Ingredients

- 1 (14 oz.) can artichoke hearts, drained and chopped
- 1 (10 oz.) package frozen chopped spinach, thawed and drained
- 1 cup mayonnaise
- 1 cup grated Parmesan cheese
- 2 1/2 cups shredded Monterey Jack cheese

## Directions

1. Preheat oven to 350 °F / 175 °C. Grease a 1-quart baking dish lightly.
2. Combine spinach, artichoke hearts, 2 cups Monterey Jack cheese, mayonnaise, and Parmesan cheese in a medium bowl. Transfer mixture to lightly greased baking dish then sprinkle with remaining 1/2 cup Monterey Jack.
3. Place the baking dish in center of preheated oven and bake for about 15 minutes until the cheese is melted.

## Nutritional Facts

Calories per serving: 211; Carbohydrates: 34g; Protein: 1g; Fat: 3g; Sugar: 1g; Sodium: 54mg; Fiber: 0g

# 34 Pinto Bean Spread

**COOKING:** 1H15'
**PREPARATION:** 15'
**SERVES:** 16

## Ingredients

- 1 (15 oz.) can pinto beans, drained and rinsed
- 1 cup nonfat cottage cheese
- 1 clove garlic
- 2 tbsps. lemon juice
- 1 tbsp. dried parsley
- 1 tsp. dried dill weed
- 1 tbsp. butter, softened
- 1/4 tsp. seasoned salt

## Directions

1. Blend seasoned salt, butter, dill, parsley, lemon juice, garlic, cottage cheese and pinto beans till smooth in blender/food processor; chill in the fridge for 1 hour minimum; serve.

## Nutritional Facts

Calories per serving: 507; Carbohydrates: 48g; Protein: 0.4g; Fat: 2g; Sugar: 0.5g; Sodium: 27mg; Fiber: 0.1g

# 35 Brownie Batter Dip

**Cooking:** 10'
**Preparation:** 10'
**Serves:** 8

## Ingredients

- 1 1/3 cups canned pinto beans
- 1/2 cup unsweetened cocoa powder
- 1/4 cup raw cashews
- 1/4 cup honey
- 2 tbsps. brown sugar
- 2 tbsps. almond milk, or more as needed
- 2 tbsps. chocolate chips

## Directions

1. Pulse brown sugar, honey, cashews, cocoa powder and pinto beans in till crumbly in a high-powered blender.
2. Add almond milk; blend till dip is smooth. Put dip in a bowl; sprinkle chocolate chips on top.

## Nutritional Facts

Calories per serving: 99; Carbohydrates: 32g; Protein: 1.7g; Fat: 2g; Sugar: 2g; Sodium: 47mg; Fiber: 0g

# Chapter 17

# Recipes:
# Vegetarian Recipes

# 36 Sirtfood Steamed Asparagus

**Cooking:** 10'
**Preparation:** 10'
**Serves:** 2

## Ingredients

- 1 bunch asparagus spears
- 1 teaspoon extra virgin olive oil
- 1/4 teaspoon sea salt
- 3 cups water

## Directions

1. Place water in the bottom half of a steamer pan set. Add salt and oil, and bring to a boil.
2. Trim the dry ends off of the asparagus. If the spears are thick, peel them lightly with a vegetable peeler. Place them in the top half of the steamer pan set. Steam for 5 to 10 minutes depending on the thickness of the asparagus, or until asparagus is tender.

**Nutritional Facts:** Calories per serving: 31; Carbohydrates: 32g; Protein: 4g; Fat: 2g; Sugar: 0.6g; Sodium: 29mg; Fiber: 1g

# 37 Sirtfood Vegetarian Quinoa and Chickpea Burger

**Cooking:** 5'
**Preparation:** 10'
**Serves:** 2

## Ingredients

- 1 1/2 cups cooked quinoa
- 2 tablespoons Dijon mustard
- 1 egg vegan (Brand: Follow Your Heart Egg Vegan), beaten
- 2 cloves garlic, minced
- 2 grinds fresh black pepper
- 1/2 cup chickpea (garbanzo bean) flour, or as needed
- 2 teaspoons olive oil, or as needed
- 2 slices gouda cheese

## Directions

1. Combine the quinoa, mustard, vegan egg, garlic, and black pepper together in a bowl; add enough chickpea flour to make 2 patties.
2. Heat oil in a pan over medium heat
3. Cook patties in oil until browned for around 4 minutes per side.
4. Add a vegan cheese slice to each patty and warm until cheese melts, about 2 and a half minutes.

## Nutritional Facts

Calories per serving: 321; Carbohydrates: 23g; Protein: 2g; Fat: 1.7g; Sugar: 1g; Sodium: 103mg; Fiber: 0g

## 38 Vegetarian Pad Thai

**Cooking:** 10'
**Preparation:** 10'
**Serves:** 2

### Ingredients

Sauce Ingredients:
- 1/2 cup honey
- 1/2 cup distilled white vinegar
- 1/4 cup soy sauce
- 2 tablespoons tamarind pulp

Main Ingredients
- 1 (12 ounce) package dried rice noodles
- 1/2 cup sesame seed oil
- 2 teaspoons minced garlic
- 4 eggs
- 1 (12 ounce) package firm tofu, cut into 1/2 inch strips
- 1 tablespoon and 1 tsp. honey
- 1 1/2 teaspoons sea salt
- 1 1/2 cups ground peanuts
- 1 1/2 teaspoons ground, dried oriental radish
- 1/2 cup chopped fresh chives
- 1 tablespoon Thai chili garlic paste
- 2 cups fresh bean sprouts
- 1 lime, cut into wedges

### Directions

1. Over medium heat combine all of the sauce ingredients.
2. Soak the rice noodles in cold water until soft and drain.
3. In a large pan, warm the olive oil, garlic and eggs over medium heat.
4. Stir to scramble the eggs.
5. Add the tofu and stir

**Nutritional Facts** — Calories per serving: 231; Carbohydrates: 42g; Protein: 0.6g; Fat: 1g; Sugar: 0.3g; Sodium: 98mg; Fiber: 1g

# 39 Farfalle with Capers

**Cooking:** 7H18'
**Preparation:** 10'
**Serves:** 4

## Ingredients

- 1 red onion, medium chopped
- 1 green bell pepper chopped
- 15 ounce can lima beans, rinsed and drained
- 15 ounce can red beans, rinsed and drained
- 28 ounce crushed tomatoes
- 1/4 cup green olives
- 2 tbsp. capers
- ½ teaspoon salt
- 1/8 teaspoon black pepper
- 2 cups vegetable stock
- 8 ounces farfalle pasta uncooked
- 1 ½ cups Vegan Cheese (Tofu Based)

<u>Garnishing Ingredients</u>

- Chopped green onions for serving

## Directions

1. Put all of the ingredients except for pasta, vegan cheese, and garnishing ingredients in your slow cooker.
2. Combine and cover.
3. Cook on high heat for 4 hours or low heat for 7 hours.
4. Add the pasta and cooking on high heat for 18 minutes, or until pasta becomes al dente
5. Add 1 cup of cheese and stir.
6. Sprinkle with the remaining vegan cheese and garnishing ingredients

## Nutritional Facts

Calories per serving: 528; Carbohydrates: 39g; Protein: 1g; Fat: 1g; Sugar: 1g; Sodium: 87mg; Fiber: 0g

## 40 Grilled Asparagus and Mushrooms

**Cooking:** 35'
**Preparation:** 10'
**Serves:** 20

### Ingredients

- 6 pcs. Crimini mushrooms, rinsed and drained
- 2 pcs. Eggplant, cut lengthwise and cut in half
- 2 pcs. Zucchini, cut lengthwise and cut in half
- 6 pcs. Asparagus

<u>Dressing Ingredients</u>

- 6 tbsp. extra virgin olive oil
- Sea salt, to taste
- 3 tbsp. apple cider vinegar
- 1 tbsp. honey
- 1 tsp. Egg-free mayonnaise

### Directions

1. Put chickpeas into Dutch oven. Cover with 14 cups of water. Bring to a boil over high heat. Reduce heat to medium and let boil for one hour.
2. Put rice and remaining water in a saucepan. Bring water to a boil and then reduce heat. Let rice cook for 14 minutes. Remove from heat and let sit 15 minutes. Fluff with a fork.
3. Cut small florets from broccoli until you have five cups.
4. Chop onion, bell pepper and celery fine.
5. Preheat oven to 375 degrees.
6. Spray a medium baking dish.
7. Steam broccoli in steamer basket for about three minutes until just tender.
8. Heat oil in skillet. Add chopped onion, bell pepper, and celery. Cook for five minutes.
9. Add cooked chickpeas, thyme, cooked rice, and broccoli. Cook for five minutes stirring constantly.
10. Put mixture into prepared baking dish.
11. Stir together remaining ingredients.
12. Pour over casserole. Bake for 30 minutes.

**Nutritional Facts**
Calories per serving: 131; Carbohydrates: 56g; Protein: 0g; Fat: 0g; Sugar: 0.4g; Sodium: 22mg; Fiber: 0g

# Chapter 18

# Recipes:
# Vegan Recipes

# 41 Vegan Broccoli and Rice Casserole

**Cooking:** 1H10'
**Preparation:** 10'
**Serves:** 4

## Ingredients

- 1 3/4 cups chickpeas
- 15 cups water, divided
- 1 1/2 cups brown rice
- 1 head broccoli
- 1 medium onion
- 1/2 red bell pepper
- 1 stalk celery
- 1 medium onion
- 1 1/4 cup unsweetened soymilk
- 1/2 cup nutritional yeast
- 4 teaspoons corn-starch
- 1 clove garlic
- 1/2 tablespoon lemon juice
- 1/2 teaspoon salt
- 1/2 teaspoon onion powder
- 1/4 teaspoon dry mustard
- 1/4 teaspoon smoked paprika
- 1/8 teaspoon cayenne pepper
- 1/4 teaspoon black pepper
- 1 teaspoon dried thyme
- Cooking spray

## Directions

1. Put chickpeas into Dutch oven. Cover with 14 cups of water. Bring to a boil over high heat. Reduce heat to medium and let boil for one hour.
2. Put rice and remaining water in a saucepan. Bring water to a boil and then reduce heat. Let rice cook for 14 minutes. Remove from heat and let sit 15 minutes. Fluff with a fork.
3. Cut small florets from broccoli until you have five cups.
4. Chop onion, bell pepper and celery fine.
5. Preheat oven to 375 degrees.
6. Spray a medium baking dish.
7. Steam broccoli in steamer basket for about three minutes until just tender.
8. Heat oil in skillet. Add chopped onion, bell pepper, and celery. Cook for five minutes.
9. Add cooked chickpeas, thyme, cooked rice, and broccoli. Cook for five minutes stirring constantly.
10. Put mixture into prepared baking dish.
11. Stir together remaining ingredients.
12. Pour over casserole. Bake for 30 minutes.

## Nutritional Facts

Calories per serving: 140; Carbohydrates: 64g; Protein: 3g; Fat: 1.3g; Sugar: 2.3g; Sodium: 17mg; Fiber: 0g

# 42 Fried Rice Pineapple

**Cooking:** 35'
**Preparation:** 10'
**Serves:** 4

## Ingredients

- 1 1/4 cups quinoa
- 1 cup water
- 1 cup organic vegetable broth
- 1/8 teaspoon salt
- 10 mini-size tofu triangles
- 1 1/2 tablespoon maple syrup, divided
- 2 teaspoons tamari
- 1 tablespoon maple syrup
- 1/8 teaspoon black pepper
- 2 red onions, divided
- 1 cup shiitake mushrooms
- 2 cups fresh pineapple, divided
- 1 cup kale
- 1/4 cup nutritional yeast
- 1/2 tsp. dried jalapeno
- 1 1/4 tablespoon mint, divided
- 3 tablespoon safflower oil
- 2 tablespoon Tahini
- 2 cups chuck pineapple
- 3 tablespoon pineapple juice

## Directions

1. Rinse quinoa in cold water and drain using a fine sieve.
2. Combine quinoa with vegetable broth and water. Bring to a boil. Cover and cook for 15 minutes.
3. Remove quinoa from heat and let sit for 15 minutes. Fluff with a fork. Set aside.
4. Dice onion.
5. Slice mushrooms.
6. Put one tablespoon safflower oil in a skillet.
7. Add tofu, sliced mushrooms and red onion and cook for one minute.
8. Add in one tablespoon maple syrup and two teaspoons tamari, and one-eighth teaspoon black pepper. Cook on high for two minutes. Flip tofu over and cook until mushrooms and onions are tender.
9. Remove tofu from pan and set aside.
10. Coarsely chop mint.
11. Add quinoa, pineapple, remaining red onion, mint, kale, nutritional yeast, jalapeno and safflower oil to red onion and mushrooms.
12. Turn heat to high and cook for three minutes.
13. Add remaining tamari and maple syrup stirring well.
14. Remove from heat and put in a bowl.
15. Add pineapple to skillet and cook until just beginning to brown.

16. In a separate bowl, combine remaining ingredients
17. Combine all ingredients stirring to combine well.
18. Add pineapple to skillet and cook until just beginning to brown.
19. In a separate bowl, combine remaining ingredients
20. Combine all ingredients stirring to combine well.

NUTRITIONAL FACTS  Calories per serving: 72; Carbohydrates: 34g; Protein: 3g; Fat: 2g; Sugar: 1g; Sodium: 20mg; Fiber: 1.4g

# 43 Sirtfood Oriental Barbecued Pork

COOKING: 8H
PREPARATION: 15'
SERVES: 4

## Ingredients

- ¼ cup of soy sauce
- ¼ cup of hoisin sauce
- 3 tablespoons of ketchup
- 3 tablespoons of honey
- 2 garlic cloves
- Small piece of fresh ginger
- 1 teaspoon of sesame oil
- ½ teaspoon of five-spice mix
- 1 boneless pork shoulder, fat trimmed
- 250ml chicken broth

## Directions

1. Crush the garlic. Peel and grate the ginger. Combine the soy sauce, hoisin sauce, ketchup, honey, crushed garlic, sesame oil and five spice powder in a bowl. Stir thoroughly.
2. Transfer the spice sauce to a seal-able plastic bag. Add the pork to the plastic bag, and then shake the bag and leave to marinate for 2 hours.
3.
4. Next, place your slow cooker onto a low setting. Empty your pork and spice sauce into the slow cooker. Cover and leave for 8 hours.
5. Finally, add the chicken broth and slow cook for another 30 minutes. Tear the pork into shreds and serve alongside the sauce.

## Nutritional Facts

Calories per serving: 654; Carbohydrates: 32g; Protein: 3g; Fat: 0.1g; Sugar: 1g; Sodium: 16mg; Fiber: 0g

# 44 Rustic French Chicken

**COOKING:** 8H'
**PREPARATION:** 15'
**SERVES:** 4

## INGREDIENTS

- 4 chicken breast halves, skinned
- 2 teaspoons dried basil
- A pinch of salt
- A pinch of black pepper
- 1 yellow bell pepper
- 400g cannellini beans
- 400g chopped tomatoes

## DIRECTIONS

1. Dice the pepper. Turn your slow cooker to a low setting and place all the ingredients in a slow cooker.
2. Cover and leave for 8 hours, then separate into four portions and serve.

**NUTRITIONAL FACTS** Calories per serving: 86; Carbohydrates: 45g; Protein: 1g; Fat: 2g; Sugar: 1g; Sodium: 87mg; Fiber: 1g

# 45 Traditional Apple Sauce

**Cooking:** 12H
**Preparation:** 25'
**Serves:** 4

## Ingredients

- ¼ cup of soy sauce
- ¼ cup of hoisin sauce
- 3 tablespoons of ketchup
- 3 tablespoons of honey
- 2 garlic cloves
- Small piece of fresh ginger
- 1 teaspoon of sesame oil
- ½ teaspoon of five-spice mix
- 1 boneless pork shoulder, fat trimmed
- 250ml chicken broth

## Directions

1. Peel the apples and chop them into large pieces. Combine the apples, spices, cider, honey and brown sugar in a slow cooker and stir.
2. Place the slow cooker on a low heat and cook for 10 hours.
3. Remove the mixture from a slow cooker. Strain the sauce through a sieve; apply pressure to any apple pieces with a spoon to extract all the juice. Remove and discard any remaining apple pulp or flesh. Return the sauce to the slow cooker and cook on low for 1 ½ hours, stirring every 10 minutes. Use as a topping for fruit and sweet treats.

## Nutritional Facts

Calories per serving: 312; Carbohydrates: 45g; Protein: 2g; Fat: 0.4g; Sugar: 2g; Sodium: 42mg; Fiber: 0g

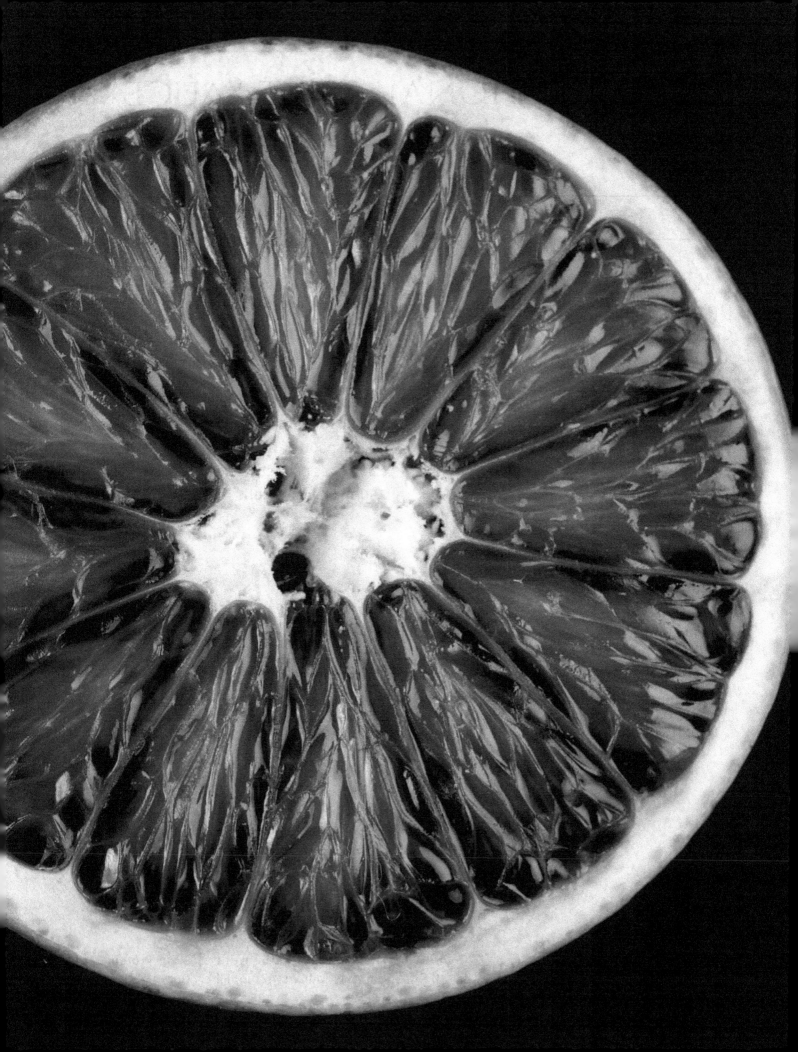

# Chapter 19

# Recipes:
# Desserts

# 46 Apricot Delight

**Cooking:** 15'
**Preparation:** 15'
**Serves:** 8

## Ingredients

- 2 cans (5-1/2 oz. each) apricot nectar, divided
- 1 package (.3 oz.) sugar-free orange gelatin
- 1 package (1 oz.) sugar-free instant vanilla pudding mix
- 2/3 cup nonfat dry milk powder
- 1 carton (8 oz.) frozen reduced-fat whipped topping, thawed
- 5 cups cubed angel food cake
- 1 can (15 oz.) reduced-sugar apricot halves, drained and sliced

## Directions

1. Add 1 cup of apricot nectar to a microwave-safe bowl and microwave for 50-60 seconds on high until hot.
2. Drizzle gelatin over hot nectar and whisk for approximately 5 minutes until the gelatin dissolves completely. Put aside to cool.
3. Mix the remaining apricot nectar with an enough amount of water in a big bowl to measure one and a quarter cups. Stir in milk powder and pudding mix for 1-2 minutes. Stir in cooled gelatin and fold in whipped topping and cake.
4. Spread over an 11x7-inch dish. Put the dish into a refrigerator for 2-4 hrs. Use apricot slices to garnish.

## Nutritional Facts

Calories per serving: 110; Carbohydrates: 12g; Protein: 4g; Fat: 2g; Sugar: 0.2g; Sodium: 43mg; Fiber: 0g

# 47 Spice Bars

**Cooking:** 45'
**Preparation:** 15'
**Serves:** 8

## Ingredients

- 3/4 cup shortening
- 3/4 cup white sugar
- 1/4 cup honey
- 1/4 cup molasses
- 2 tsps. baking soda
- 1 tsp. ground cinnamon
- 1 tsp. ground ginger
- 1/2 tsp. ground cloves
- 2 1/2 cups all-purpose flour
- 3/4 cup raisins (optional)
- 1 cup confectioners' sugar
- 3 tbsps. milk
- 1/2 tsp. vanilla extract

## Directions

1. Preheat the oven to 175°C or 350°Fahrenheit. Lightly oil a 9-in x 13-in baking dish.
2. Cream shortening and white sugar together in a medium bowl; fold in honey and molasses. Sieve cloves, flour, baking soda, ginger, and cinnamon together. Mix flour mixture and creamed mixture together until well combined; fold in raisins.
3. Evenly spread the batter in the baking dish. Bake in the preheated oven for 20-30mins until golden brown and the surface is dry and smooth to the touch.
4. For the icing, combine vanilla, milk, and confectioners' sugar together in a smaller bowl. Spread icing over the warm spice bars; cool. Cut bars then serve.

## Nutritional Facts

Calories per serving: 167; Carbohydrates: 16g; Protein: 1g; Fat: 0g; Sugar: 0.6g; Sodium: 36mg; Fiber: 0g

# 48 Sirtfood Pretzel Strawberry Dessert

**Cooking:** 30'
**Preparation:** 30'
**Serves:** 18

## Ingredients

- 2-2/3 cups crushed pretzels (10 oz.)
- 1 cup butter, melted
- 1 package (8 oz.) cream cheese, softened
- 1 cup sugar
- 1 carton (8 oz.) frozen whipped topping, thawed
- 1 can (20 oz.) crushed pineapple
- 2 packages (3 oz. each) strawberry gelatin
- 2 packages (10 oz. each) frozen sliced sweetened strawberries, thawed

## Directions

1. Combine butter and pretzels in a bowl. Press onto the bottom of an oiled baking dish, about 13x9 inches. Bake at 350° until set, about 8 to 10 minutes. Place on wire rack to cool. Beat sugar and cream cheese in a bowl until they become smooth.
2. Then fold in the whipped topping and spread over the cooled crust. Place in the refrigerator until chilled.
3. Drain the pineapple, saving the juice; put pineapple aside. If necessary, pour water into pineapple juice to measure one cup; mix into the gelatin mixture. Place in the refrigerator until set partially. Mix in the strawberries and reserved pineapple. Spoon over the filling carefully. Refrigerate, covered, until firm, about 3 to 4 hours.

## Nutritional Facts

Calories per serving: 423; Carbohydrates: 38g; Protein: 1g; Fat: 1.6g; Sugar: 0g; Sodium: 80mg; Fiber: 0g

# 49 Sirtfood Cherry Cheescake Pie

**Cooking:** 10'
**Preparation:** 10'
**Serves:** 8

## Ingredients

- 1 (9 inch) prepared graham cracker crust
- 1 (8 oz.) package cream cheese, softened
- 1 (14 oz.) can sweetened condensed milk
- 1 (21 oz.) can cherry pie filling, chilled
- 1/2 cup lemon juice
- 1 tsp. vanilla extract

## Directions

1. Beat cream cheese till fluffy in a medium bowl.
2. Add condensed milk; thoroughly mix. Mix in vanilla and lemon juice.
3. Put into crust. Chill for 2 hours. Before serving, top with cherry/other pie filling. Refrigerate.

## Nutritional Facts

Calories per serving: 221; Carbohydrates: 16g; Protein: 2g; Fat: 2g; Sugar: 0.4g; Sodium: 120mg; Fiber: 0.7g

# 50 Fluffy Orange Gelatin Pie

**Cooking:** 15'
**Preparation:** 15'
**Serves:** 8

## Ingredients

- 1 can (15 oz.) mandarin oranges
- 1 package (3 oz.) orange gelatin
- 1 can (5 oz.) evaporated milk, chilled
- 1 reduced-fat graham cracker crust (8 inches)
- 1 medium navel orange, sliced

## Directions

1. Drain the liquid from the oranges to measuring cup. Put enough water to measure one cup; put the oranges aside.
2. Add liquid to the saucepan; boil. Whisk in gelatin till dissolved.
3. Move into big bowl; add the mixer beaters into the bowl. Keep covered and refrigerated till the mixture is syrupy.
4. Put in the milk. Beat on high speed till almost doubled. Fold in the mandarin oranges. Add to the crust. Keep in the refrigerator till becoming set, 2 to 3 hours. Use the slices of the orange to decorate.

## Nutritional Facts

Calories per serving: 543; Carbohydrates: 20g; Protein: 1g; Fat: 3g; Sugar: 2g; Sodium: 34mg; Fiber: 1g

# Chapter 19

# Recipes:
# Green Juice

# 51 Sirtfood Minty Green Juice

**Cooking:** 0
**Preparation:** 10'
**Serves:** 2

## Ingredients

- 1 1/2 oz. of baby spinach
- 4 oz. of pineapple (chopped)
- 1 apple (chopped)
- 1 handful of mint (stemmed)
- 1 tablespoon of hemp seeds
- 2 tablespoons of coconut water
- a pinch of sea salt
- 1 cup of ice

## Directions

1. Place all ingredients in a blender putting the leafy vegetables last. Add a little more water if you prefer a smoother consistency.
2. Process until thoroughly blended.
3. Shake it up or stir it up. For garnish you can use, lemon, celery, slice of tomato and chia seeds. Add ice if you prefer it cold. Serve and enjoy.

## Nutritional Facts

Calories per serving: 104; Carbohydrates: 24.1g; Protein: 2g; Fat: 0.4g; Sugar: 1g; Sodium: 103mg; Fiber: 1.2g

# 52 Sirtfood Persimmon-Mint Magic

COOKING: 0
PREPARATION: 10'
SERVES: 2

## Ingredients

- 1 1/2 oz. of collard greens
- 1 apple (chopped)
- 1 persimmon (topped)
- 3 sprigs of mint
- 1 teaspoon of matcha tea
- 1 cup of water
- 1 cup of ice

## Directions

1. 1 1/2 oz. of collard greens
2. 1 apple (chopped)
3. 1 persimmon (topped)
4. 3 sprigs of mint
5. 1 teaspoon of matcha tea
6. 1 cup of water
7. 1 cup of ice
8. Directions:
9. Place all ingredients in a blender putting the leafy vegetables last. Add a little more water if you prefer a smoother consistency.
10. Process until thoroughly blended.
11. Shake it up or you can stir it. For garnish you can use, lemon, celery, slice of tomato and chia seeds. Add ice if you prefer it cooler. Serve and enjoy.

## Nutritional Facts

Calories per serving: 311; Carbohydrates: 49.6g; Protein: 2g; Fat: 0.4g; Sugar: 0g; Sodium: 61mg; Fiber: 1g

# 53 Sirtfood Pears N' Spinach

**Cooking:** 0
**Preparation:** 15'
**Serves:** 2

## Ingredients

- 1 1/2 oz. of baby spinach
- 1 apple (chopped)
- 1 pear (chopped)
- 1 teaspoon of cinnamon
- 1 tablespoon of flaxseeds
- 1 cup of water
- 1 cup of ice

## Directions

1. Place all ingredients in a blender putting the leafy vegetables last. Add a little more water if you prefer a smoother consistency.
2. Process until thoroughly blended.
3. Shake it up or stir it up. For garnish you can use, lemon, celery, slice of tomato and chia seeds. Add ice if you prefer it cooler. Serve and enjoy.

## Nutritional Facts

Calories per serving: 164; Carbohydrates: 33g; Protein: 1.4g; Fat: 2g; Sugar: 0.3g; Sodium: 43mg; Fiber: 1g

# 54 Sirtfood Protein Green

**Cooking:** 0
**Preparation:** 15'
**Serves:** 2

## Ingredients

- 1 1/2 oz. baby spinach
- 2 clementine's (peeled and pegged)
- 1 apple (chopped)
- 1 tablespoon of flaxseeds
- 1 tablespoon of pea protein
- 1 cup of water
- 1 cup of ice

## Directions

1. Place all ingredients in a blender putting the leafy vegetables last. Add a little more water if you prefer a smoother consistency.
2. Process until thoroughly blended.
3. Shake it up or stir it up. For garnish you can use, lemon, celery, a slice of tomato and chia seeds. Add ice if you prefer it cold. Serve and enjoy.

## Nutritional Facts

Calories per serving: 118; Carbohydrates: 65g; Protein: 1.8g; Fat: 2g; Sugar: 0.3g; Sodium: 72mg; Fiber: 0g

# 55 Sirtfood Sunflower Spinach

**Cooking:** 0
**Preparation:** 15'
**Serves:** 2

## Ingredients

- 1 1/2 oz. of baby spinach
- 1 banana (peeled)
- 1 tablespoon of sunflower seeds
- 1 teaspoon of cinnamon
- 1 cup of water
- 1 cup of ice

## Directions

1. Wash and chop vegetables.
2. Place all ingredients in a blender putting the spinach last. Add a little more water if you prefer a smoother consistency. Process until thoroughly blended.
3. Shake it up or stir it up. For garnish you can use, lemon, celery, a slice of tomato and chia seeds. Add ice if you prefer it cold. Serve and enjoy.

## Nutritional Facts

Calories per serving: 330; Carbohydrates: 54g; Protein: 1.2g; Fat: 1g; Sugar: 0.4g; Sodium: 86mg; Fiber: 0g

# CONCLUSION

With all the food regimen fads that have considering popped out from nowhere, people have been trying their first-rate to get to the lowest of it all. Many of us need to realize which program offers high-quality results and provide overall benefits. Is there something that offers long time blessings at all?

The Sirtfood Diet is all about consuming the right foods and getting fast consequences. It is the maximum popular eating regimen to date, ably overturning outcomes that made the Dukan and Paleo famous. This food plan entails meals with large quantities of Sirtuin activators.

These activators switch on the body's skinny gene pathways by way of approach of exercising and fasting for you to burn fats, enhance muscles, and beautify fitness. The diet regime includes meals and advice that might maintain you off from the burden you lost all through the first week of this system and integrating extra Sirtfoods to your meals as you go along.

With around 650 million overweight adults around the world, it's crucial to find healthful meals and doable exercising programs, don't throw away the whole thing you love and don't must exercise all the time. Time. Week. The Sirtfood weight loss program does just that: The idea is that certain meals set off the "lean gene" pathways that are generally activated by way of fasting and workout.

As soon as the weight loss program becomes a way of life during exercising, it is critical to eat protein one hour after a workout preferably. The protein repairs muscles after exercising, relieve ache, and can sell regeneration. There are loads of recipes that include proteins best for post-exercise consumption, e.g., For example, B. Sirt Chili con Carne or turmeric-chicken-kale salad. If you want something lighter, you can attempt the Sirt Blueberry smoothie and upload protein powder for extra benefits. The type of health you exercise is up to you. However, in case you are educated at home, you could pick while you want to exercise, what sorts of sporting events are right for you, and are quick and convenient.

Take note that you should maintain the weight loss results through Phase 2 and continue to lose weight gradually. Also, the one striking thing we've seen with the Sirtfood Diet is that most or all of the weight people lose is from fat and that many put some muscle on. So, we would like to warn you again not to measure your success solely based on the numbers. Look in the mirror to see if you look leaner and more toned, see how well your clothes fit and lap up the compliments you'll get from others.

The Sirtfood diet is a first-rate way to trade your consuming habits, lose weight, and experience healthier. The first few weeks may be difficult. However, it's critical to test which meals are high-quality to devour and which delicious recipes are proper for you. Be type to yourself for the first few weeks, as your body adapts and trains while you need to. If you are already exercising moderately or intensively, you'll be able to preserve as standard or manipulate your health primarily based on the exchange in diet. As with any change in food plan and workout, it all depends on the individual and what kind of effort you can make.

I hope you have learned something!

CPSIA information can be obtained
at www.ICGtesting.com
Printed in the USA
LVHW061639181020
669109LV00034B/978